Beyond the Footprints of Menopause

by Sheila Whitener, RN, MSN, CCM

ISBN: [979-8-218-79994-6]

Published by Sheila Whitener

Disclaimer:

This book is for informational purposes only and is not intended as a substitute for medical advice. Always consult with a qualified healthcare professional before making any changes to your health, diet, or wellness regimen.

First and foremost, I give thanks to God for guiding me through this journey and for giving me the strength and inspiration to complete this book. I also want to thank my Husband, my mother, my sons, and my siblings for encouraging me to keep pursuing my dreams and never giving up.

Table of Contents

Introduction...

Chapter 1: Understanding the Shift: How Hormones Shape Our Bodies and Minds 9

Chapter 2: The Emotional Weight We Carry 30

Chapter 3: The Other Half of the Story: The Physical Weight We Carry 63

Chapter 4: The Spiritual Journey...........................83

Chapter 5: Carrying the Healing Forward..................107

Chapter 6: Soul Nourishment................................126

Chapter 7: Confidence in the Mirror 145

Chapter 8: Redefining Intimacy 168

Chapter 9: Embracing the Best Version of You 192

Chapter 10: Too Old for What? To Stop Becoming? Not a Chance...213

Chapter 11: The Ripple Effect: When Your Light Touches Others 231

Chapter 12: The End of This Chapter: The Next One Is Yours to Write...250

Closing Poem: From My Heart to Yours 264

Introduction

Each footprint in the sand reflects a step through the journey of menopause—a challenge confronted, an obstacle overcome, a moment of resilience. Some imprints are deep, shaped by hormonal shifts, restless nights, and the emotional weight of change, while others are lighter, filled with newfound confidence and the strength to move forward. Yet with each step, we redefine what it means to thrive, embracing this journey with grace and vitality.

I remember when menopause changed everything— my body, my emotions, my confidence. I traveled to some very dark places. The hot flashes every 5 minutes, the mood swings, the anxiety attacks. As I began this challenging journey, life threw even more obstacles my way. I kept asking God, how am I going to make it through? How can I take back control of my life? In time, I realized this was not the end at all; it was an awakening, a breaking point that became my breakthrough, guiding me towards a version of myself that I did not yet know existed. After all these years, I am finally stepping into the confidence I have never known before. The truth is, some of the most beautiful transformations happen after we have been broken.

While there were moments when I felt isolated, unsure, and overwhelmed, I also knew that there were other countless women who were also navigating this transition, searching for strength, clarity, and reassurance. Menopause is more than a physical transition—it's an emotional awakening as well. The doubts, the shifts, the moments of uncertainty, they do not define you. This is your time to rediscover your strength, embrace your self-worth, and step into a confidence that is wholly, unapologetically yours. The emotional journey of menopause is not about losing yourself; it is about rediscovering and embracing the powerful, radiant woman you have always been.

I have faced the challenges, felt the weight of uncertainty, but have discovered the strategies that turned surviving into thriving. I will share with you how I reclaimed my self-worth and found peace in this new chapter of my life. I am here to help you navigate your future footprints- so that you can reclaim your confidence, embrace your self-worth, and step into this chapter of your life with unwavering strength and power. This is not just about following a path; it is about creating new footprints for yourself, walking in your truth, and thriving through this season with confidence, self-love, and the best version of you. The purpose of this book is to inspire those who feel as if they have left no footprints behind—those quietly journeying through life, wondering if their path matters. It is a powerful reminder that every step holds meaning and that it is never too late to blaze a trail. With heartfelt motivation and unwavering encouragement, this book is a beacon for anyone searching for the strength to keep going and the belief that their story deserves to be told.

This book is about reclaiming the parts of yourself that menopause tried to silence. It is about navigating the emotional ups and downs, rediscovering your self-image, rebuilding your sense of self-worth, and stepping boldly into a new season of confidence. It is a guide for every woman ready to stop merely surviving menopause and start thriving emotionally, mentally, and unapologetically. This book is for every woman on her menopause journey, who is prepared to find healing, strength, and self-love.

May this book meet you where you are and gently lead you to where your soul has longed to go. With every page, may you feel more seen, more rooted, more whole. This journey is for you—the real you. Come as you are. You are enough.

CHAPTER 1

Understanding the Shift

How Hormones Shape Our Bodies and Minds

1 *Understanding the Shift: How Hormones Shape Our Bodies and Minds*

Before we can fully step into the journey of thriving through menopause, it is important to understand what's happening inside our bodies during this transition. Too often, women are expected to endure the changes without real explanations, leaving them feeling frustrated, confused, and overwhelmed by symptoms they didn't see coming. I believe that knowledge is one of the most powerful tools a woman can have in this season of her life. By understanding the physiological changes of menopause—how your hormones affect your body, mind, and emotions—you gain insight into why you feel different, and you will be able to respond with clarity and compassion instead of reacting blindly. Yes, compassion is loving yourself, listening gently to your body's whispers, honoring your emotional tides, and standing in the truth of your transformation.

Let's take a moment to review the inner shifts your body undergoes during menopause. Having a clear understanding of the hormonal and physical changes equips you to recognize what's normal, when to seek support, and how to respond in ways that nurture your whole self. This chapter is not here to overwhelm you with information or medical jargon; it is about giving you the essential knowledge every woman deserves so you can feel informed, confident, and in control of her own journey.

All women cross into this sacred season of menopause, where transformation quietly unfolds. We may not have the same symptoms; some of us may have extreme symptoms, while others will experience only mild ones, but we will all reach this season in our lives. Though you may hear women say they have never gone through menopause, this is often a misunderstanding. In truth, every woman who journeys far enough in life enters this season—a quiet rite of passage woven into the rhythm of womanhood. Menopause is a natural biological process, not something you can bypass. This hormonal shift takes place in every woman's body, whether she openly recognizes it or not.

Clarifying the truths behind hormonal changes during menopause matters deeply—because when we make space for honest conversation of why our bodies go through these changes, women are free to walk this path with confidence and self-trust, not isolation or misplaced shame. Many women walk through this season carrying physical and emotional shifts in their bodies, unaware that these changes are part of what we call "the transformation." This is why I emphasize again that education is the starting point. The key to recognizing those whispers and beginning to truly listen—is daring to pause long enough to hear your soul and body speak.

Understanding the Hormonal Landscape of Menopause

Much like shifting gears in a car, the hormonal shift demands adjustment: sometimes smooth, sometimes jolting. It's the body recalibrating, finding a new rhythm, and learning how to operate in a different mode. The key is understanding the mechanics behind this shift so you can navigate the ride with confidence.

You may also hear the phrase that we are at war with our hormones, but I see it differently. We are not at war with our hormones when they're not willing to stay and fight. They are leaving us—shifting, pulling away. If anything, we are left longing for their presence, knowing we must adjust to the changes they leave behind as they fade. It is truly not a war; it is a shift, and one we must learn to navigate. How can we fully grasp the changes we're experiencing if we are not informed about the connection between our reproductive system and hormones? Let's take a moment to reflect on the changes our bodies undergo during this hormonal shift, and the powerful role hormones play in driving this transition.

Let's take it from the beginning—I mean from the very beginning. When women are born, we are born with all the eggs we're going to have for the rest of our lives. A developing fetus with ovaries initially has about 6 to 7 million eggs. When we are born, we have about 1 to 2 million eggs. The reproductive system—more specifically, the ovaries—does not make any more eggs. By the time puberty hits, many of these eggs start to disintegrate and are reabsorbed into the body. The eggs that are left are waiting to be fertilized. These eggs mature over time, and somewhere between the ages of twelve and older, our eggs are ready for fertilization by a male's sperm. (They're probably backstage bickering over who gets the first pick of the next handsome catch!) Now, of course, there are cases where pregnancy has happened at an even earlier age.

The Relationship Between the Ovaries, the Eggs, and the Hormones

Beyond serving as a home for these eggs, the ovaries are responsible for producing estrogen, a key hormone that regulates the menstrual cycle and ensures eggs mature properly. Estrogen helps stimulate the growth of ovarian follicles, creating ideal conditions for egg development. It also prepares the uterus for possible implantation, supporting overall fertility. Other hormones like testosterone and progesterone also play a role in the shift, but estrogen is the primary driver. As hormonal shifts occur—especially during menopause—the ovaries gradually reduce their estrogen production. When estrogen takes that dive, the eggs can no longer mature, and again, the eggs disintegrate. Just think, they were waiting all that time to get fertilized, and it never happened. They did not get a chance to meet their handsome prince. Remember, we do not lose all our estrogen. Other organs in the body, such as the adrenal glands, still produce small amounts, but the ovaries remain the primary producers.

Menopause Unveiled: The Hormonal Shifts Across Its Three Phases

Hormonal shifts can lead to significant physical and emotional changes. The mood swings, the hot flashes, the weight gain, the thinning of the hair—I could go on and on about the shift in our bodies because every shift carries a story worth telling. Change begins with the quiet drop of hormone levels.

The changes can start in your forties, and for some, even sooner. This is called the perimenopausal phase. In the perimenopause phase, hormones start to fluctuate and decline, and some women will have mild to moderate symptoms. These symptoms can be similar to those in menopause—like hot flashes, mood swings, and brain fog. However, some women in their forties may not realize these symptoms are signs of perimenopause, or they may not want to consider that possibility at all. You might hear some women insist, "I'm way too young for menopause symptoms," and trust me, they're not looking for a response. At that moment, silence is your safest strategy.

The next phase is called the menopause phase. This is a natural stage marking the end of menstruation, officially diagnosed after 12 consecutive months without a period. So, you see, the actual menopausal phase does not last that long. Once you miss your period for twelve consecutive months, this marks the end of your menopause phase.

The next phase for the rest of your life is the postmenopausal phase, which is hardly ever brought up—everyone says "menopause," yet postmenopausal is left out. For some women, whether menopause or post-menopause, the label does not matter. Regardless of the phase, most women focus on the symptoms and shifts, but it's equally important to understand each phase. So, let's review this again in simpler terms: Hormones fluctuate in perimenopause → symptoms start. A big crash happens (the hormones take a dive), and menopause → symptoms often peak. Post-menopause → estrogen stays low → some symptoms ease, but others (like vaginal dryness, bone loss, and sleep problems) can persist if untreated.

The postmenopausal phase is when women are more at risk for chronic conditions such as heart disease, high blood pressure, and diabetes. The reason? Hormones are at their lowest and can no longer protect the body. Estrogen helps make blood vessels elastic and strong. When estrogen diminishes, arteries become stiffer and narrower.

No Two Journeys Are the Same: The Wide Range of Menopause Symptoms

There is another myth or misconception that symptoms of menopause will eventually disappear— like hot flashes, mood swings, and brain fog—but the truth is that for some, these symptoms can linger for many years. Why the difference? Genetics, body composition, overall health, and stress management levels all play a role. They can become less severe over time or as the woman continues to age.

I was one of those women who experienced very severe symptoms, starting with hot flashes every 5 minutes. I would have an aura right before my hot flash with the feeling of dizziness and as though I was going to faint. I thought something was seriously wrong until I started to notice a pattern. I was in the emergency room at least 3–4 times a year because I was not sure at first if there was something more serious going on.

With years of experience as a Registered Nurse, staying attentive to my health has always been a priority. Truth be told, even nurses are not immune to a touch of hypochondria from time to time. I like to say that whenever you're uncertain about what's happening, and whether your symptoms are due to menopause, never assume—always seek medical advice first, because it could be something more serious.

I finally realized that the symptoms I was having were part of my menopausal phase—or should I say, my postmenopausal phase.

While menopause and post-menopause are often associated with a variety of challenging symptoms, it's important to recognize that not every woman experiences this transition the same way. Again, as I stated earlier, some women will glide through menopause with very few noticeable symptoms or discomfort. Knowing that experiencing a milder symptom journey is completely normal can provide reassurance and help break the myth that menopause is always difficult for every woman.

The Link Between Hysterectomy and Menopausal Symptoms

A total hysterectomy, which is the surgical removal of the uterus and cervix, does not have an impact on a woman's menopausal journey—but the effects depend on whether the ovaries are removed during the hysterectomy. If the ovaries remain intact with the total hysterectomy, a woman may continue to produce hormones like estrogen and progesterone, and menopausal symptoms will typically begin naturally at its usual time. If you have a total hysterectomy, which again is the removal of the cervix and uterus along with the removal of both ovaries (called a bilateral oophorectomy causes immediate menopause symptoms. This is often referred to as induced or surgical menopause. This sudden drop in hormone levels can lead to more abrupt and intense menopausal symptoms compared to a natural menopause transition. A partial hysterectomy removes the upper part of the uterus and preserves the cervix. Again, this can be accompanied by removing the ovaries or leaving the ovaries in place. If ovaries are left in place, menopausal symptoms should happen naturally. Whether or not your physician decides to remove your ovaries depends on what type of condition the ovaries are in. Understanding this connection is important for women who have had, or are going to have, a hysterectomy, so they can prepare for how it might influence their hormonal health. Every woman needs to have a conversation with their physician and understand what is being removed, because far too many women go through procedures like a hysterectomy without fully knowing what was removed from their bodies. In talking with countless women over the years, I was surprised by how many women were not sure if they still had their cervix or if it was removed, or if their ovaries, whether one or both, were left in place. It is also good to know if there was one ovary removed, was it the right ovary or the left ovary? This information does matter. It matters because what's removed affects your hormones, your menopause journey, and your long-term health.

How Menopause Shifts Fat Storage to the Midsection

There are countless shifts our bodies go through during menopause, but in this chapter, I will focus on a few of the most important ones. While it's impossible to cover everything here, I dive much deeper into these changes and how to manage these changes inside Menopause Energized, my signature coaching program. As women move through menopause, one of the most common and frustrating changes is unexpected weight gain—particularly around the midsection. This is not just about overeating or lack of exercise; it's largely driven by hormonal shifts, especially the drop in estrogen. Estrogen plays a role in how and where the body stores fat, and when estrogen levels decline, the body tends to store excessive fat deep in the abdominal cavity, known as visceral fat.

Unlike the fat that sits just beneath the skin, visceral fat surrounds your internal organs like the liver, pancreas, and intestines. This type of fat is especially concerning because it's metabolically active and can increase the risk of heart disease, type 2 diabetes, and inflammation in the body. Even women who maintain the same diet and activity level they had before may still notice stubborn belly weight due to these internal changes. Therefore, as our bodies shift during menopause, so must our habits—because transformation calls for partnership, not resistance. Understanding this connection allows women to approach midlife weight management with more self-compassion and smarter, hormone-friendly strategies—rather than guilt or extreme dieting.

Hormonal Shifts and Heart Health

One important but often overlooked change during menopause is the effect on heart health. Many women don't realize that estrogen has played a quiet, protective role for their cardiovascular system.

Estrogen helps maintain healthy cholesterol levels, keeps blood vessels flexible, and supports overall circulation. It also helps regulate blood pressure and reduce inflammation in the arteries. As estrogen levels decline during menopause, this natural protection fades, and the risk for cardiovascular issues—including high blood pressure, heart disease, and stroke—begins to rise. In fact, heart disease is the leading health risk for women after menopause. What makes this even more concerning is that menopausal symptoms like weight gain, increased visceral fat, sleep disturbances, and higher stress levels can also contribute to cardiovascular strain. Many women notice changes in their cholesterol numbers and blood pressure during this transition, sometimes without obvious warning signs.

That is why understanding this connection is important; it empowers women to be proactive about their heart health, making intentional choices regarding nutrition, physical activity, stress management, and regular health screenings. By staying informed and paying attention to these shifts, women can take meaningful steps to protect their hearts and overall well-being throughout their menopausal years.

How Hormones Influence Mood and Emotional Well-Being

One of the most noticeable—and sometimes unexpected—changes women experience during menopause is the emotional shift that comes with fluctuating hormone levels. Estrogen directly influences key brain chemicals like serotonin, which helps regulate mood, emotional balance, and a sense of well-being. As estrogen declines, so does its steady effect on these neurotransmitters, which can lead to increased irritability, anxiety, sadness, and mood swings. Many women report feeling more emotionally sensitive, reactive, or unsettled during this time, even if they have never struggled with mood issues before. This is a very real, physical response to shifting hormones—not a character flaw or weakness. Additionally, midlife often brings its own set of emotional triggers, including children leaving home, aging parents, career transitions, relationship changes, and confronting one's own aging process. These life events, coupled with hormonal changes, can

amplify feelings of being overwhelmed, insecure, and frustrated. Emotional resilience can feel harder to maintain when your body's natural mood-regulating system is out of balance.

This is why understanding this connection is so important. Recognizing that these emotional ups and downs are part of the hormonal shift, which allows women to approach themselves with more compassion and seek out tools, support, and practices that can ease the emotional weight of this season. This is discussed in more detail in the next chapter.

Moving Forward

This chapter is only the beginning of the true shift of menopause. While countless changes are happening beneath the surface, learning about these core changes gives you a solid foundation to build upon. You deserve to move through menopause feeling informed, supported, and empowered—not lost in a storm of symptoms you don't understand. Remember, this transition is not meant to break you; it is meant to awaken you with clarity and care, so you can navigate this journey with strength, grace, and renewed purpose. The first step in handling this shift is acknowledging it—giving yourself permission to feel what you're feeling without guilt, shame, or the pressure to push through like nothing's happening. Begin by paying attention to your body and emotions, noticing patterns and changes, and trusting that these shifts are a natural part of your life's journey. From there, educate yourself about what's happening within your body, and don't hesitate to seek out resources, support groups, or healthcare professionals who truly listen and understand this season.

Simple changes in daily habits—like nourishing your body with hormone-supportive foods, finding movement that feels good, prioritizing rest, and practicing mindfulness—can make a real difference. Most importantly, extend grace to yourself along the way. This is not a race to "fix" everything, but an opportunity to reconnect with your body, advocate for your needs, and care for yourself in ways you may have long neglected.

Conclusion

As women, our bodies are constantly evolving, but the hormonal shifts of menopause marks one of the most profound transitions we'll experience in our lifetime. These changes don't just affect our physical health; they touch every part of us—from our emotions and sleep to our relationships and sense of identity.

Understanding the details of your own body is not just about knowing medical facts. It's about using that knowledge to take action, reclaim ownership of your health, and make informed, empowered decisions moving forward. This understanding also shapes how you manage your wellness, hormone support, and preventative care in the years ahead.

By understanding what's happening within our bodies during this season, we begin to remove the fear, shame, and confusion that often surround menopause. Knowledge is more than just power; it is peace of mind. When you can name what you are going through and why it's happening, you reclaim control over your body, your choices, and your emotional well-being.

The first step in navigating this hormonal shift is acknowledging your feelings without judgment and tuning into your body's changes. Educate yourself, seek support, and approach this transition with patience and self-compassion. By doing so, you open the door to healing, growth, and a more empowered, vibrant next chapter.

This chapter is only the beginning of true awareness. While countless shifts are happening beneath the surface, learning about these core changes gives you a solid foundation to build upon. You deserve to move through menopause feeling informed, supported, and empowered—not lost in a storm of symptoms you don't understand. Beyond the Footprints of

Menopause is your invitation to walk with wisdom, not fear.

Affirmation: *"I honor my body and emotions. I tune in to what my body is telling me. I honor my symptoms as messengers, educate myself with compassion, and take action that supports my transformation."*

Chapter 2

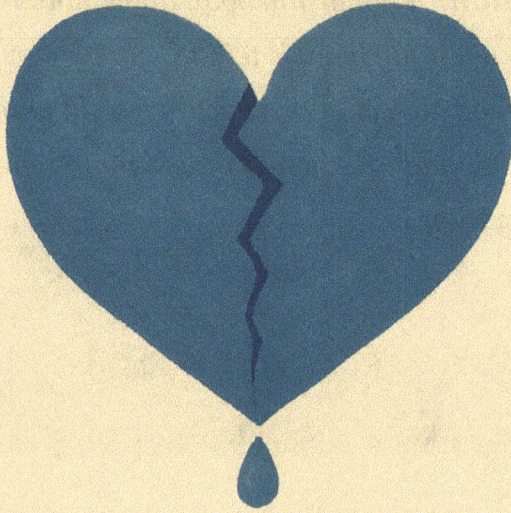

The Emotional Weight We Carry

2 The Emotional Weight We Carry

This chapter dives into the unhealed emotional baggage, old insecurities, grief, and unresolved feelings that often surface during menopause. As the body undergoes significant changes, it's common for buried emotions and past wounds to rise to the surface, demanding attention and healing. Menopause is not just a physical transition — it's a profound emotional journey that can bring forgotten pain back into focus. These feelings may feel overwhelming or confusing, but they also offer an opportunity for gentle reflection and release. In this chapter, we will explore how to recognize these resurfacing emotions, understand their origins, and approach them with kindness and patience. By learning how to unpack and heal this emotional baggage gently, you can create space for renewed peace, self-compassion, and emotional freedom on your menopause journey.

Breaking the Silence: Why Menopause Remains a Hidden Conversation

Menopause continues to be a taboo subject in many cultures and societies because of its challenges and long-held beliefs about aging, femininity, and women's roles. Unlike other life stages that are openly discussed and even celebrated, menopause is often shrouded in silence, embarrassment, or misinformation. This silence stems from societal discomfort with aging women and the physical and emotional changes they experience, leading to stigma and misunderstanding. Many women feel isolated because they lack open conversations, education, and support around menopause. The result is a culture where menopause is hidden rather than embraced, making it harder for women to seek the help and resources they need during this significant life transition. Why is it that even in households, women are embarrassed to talk about their symptoms with their husbands, and the husbands are too embarrassed to ask? I don't think society truly understands what this shift is in a woman's life. Too often, it's dismissed as an excuse or brushed off as if women are just complaining. But unless someone has walked this path, it's impossible to fully grasp what it feels like — physically, emotionally, and mentally. Even those who have experienced menopause often struggle to explain the changes happening within their own bodies and minds.

The taboo surrounding menopause deepens the emotional struggle many women face during this transition. When society avoids open conversations about menopause, it leaves women feeling isolated, misunderstood, and hesitant to share their experiences. This silence can amplify feelings of shame, anxiety, and loneliness, making it harder to cope with the emotional ups and downs that menopause brings. Without education and support, women may blame themselves for mood swings or emotional challenges instead of recognizing them as natural parts of this phase. Breaking the taboo is essential—not only to provide accurate information but to create a compassionate space where women feel seen, heard, and empowered to navigate their emotions with confidence.

Breaking the silence around menopause is a vital step towards healing the emotional turmoil many women face during this transition. When we openly talk about menopause, sharing our experiences, challenges, and truths, we create a supportive community that validates feelings often dismissed or misunderstood. This openness helps women realize they are not alone, which reduces isolation and shame. Education and honest conversations empower women to recognize that their emotions are natural responses, not personal weaknesses. By breaking the taboo, we foster compassion and understanding, encouraging women to seek the support and resources they need. This collective voice becomes a powerful force, transforming menopause from a hidden struggle into a shared journey of strength and resilience.

Struggling With Our Emotions During Menopause

One of the biggest challenges women face during menopause is the struggle to manage their emotions. When our emotions feel out of control, everything else in life feels out of balance as well. The truth is, you can't truly thrive through menopause until you learn how to take charge of your emotional well-being.

Menopause deeply affects the emotional landscape of a woman's life. The hormonal fluctuations that occur during this time impact neurotransmitters in the brain, which regulates mood, sleep, and stress response. This biological shift can make emotions feel more intense, unpredictable, and harder to manage than before. On top of that, menopause often coincides with other life stressors—such as aging parents, career pressures, or changes in relationships—that add to the emotional burden. Many women find themselves navigating feelings of loss, uncertainty, and frustration, sometimes without the support or understanding they need. This complex mix of physical changes and life challenges creates a perfect storm that makes the emotional journey through menopause uniquely difficult for many.

Let's talk about stress and anxiety. As women, we already bear a great deal of weight — spouses, aging parents, and caring for our children if we had them later in life. Then menopause arrives, often hitting us like a ton of bricks. The hardest part is that no one around truly understands what we are hit with. Life still demands what you can do for them, while you're silently battling emotional turmoil on the inside, wishing you could scream.

The truth is that most people are not educated about the menopause journey or the invisible struggles some of us face. They don't recognize the weight we have to carry. You show up for everyone else, but who shows up for you? That's when isolation creeps in. You start to feel like you have nowhere to turn, because to others, it might just look like you're being too emotional. So, where do you go? Who truly understands? That's the reality for too many women today — and it is exactly why conversations like this matter.

The Emotional Roller Coaster Ride

Menopause takes you on an emotional roller coaster you never signed up for, but you get to decide how the ride ends. Every dip, turn, and loop on this emotional roller coaster reveals a woman rediscovering her voice, her power, and her peace. Some days you're soaring high, and other days you're barely holding on; that's the wild emotional ride of menopause. It is a ride with no map, no seatbelt, and no warning signs, but you're stronger than every twist and turn. The emotional roller coaster ride is not here to break you; it's here to show you what you're made of. You can scream, cry, laugh, or throw your hands up because this ride belongs to you now. One minute you are happy, and the next minute you are sad. Does any of this sound familiar? The back and forth was driving me absolutely crazy, and my husband could not understand what was going on with me. Then you start blaming yourself, wondering if something is wrong with you. But instead of just saying it is those frustrating hormones, we need to truly understand what's happening inside our bodies and why our emotions can feel so overwhelming.

Estrogen's Role in Mood Regulation

It is not just in your head; it is in your brain chemistry. During menopause, the drop in estrogen alters how your brain processes emotions, stress, and resilience. This is why some days feel like an emotional roller coaster you never bought a ticket for. Understanding the why behind those ups and downs can give you the power to manage the ride on your terms. Estrogen is not just about reproductive health; it is a powerful neuromodulator in the brain. It interacts with serotonin, dopamine, and norepinephrine, which are brain chemicals that regulate mood, stress response, and emotional

balance. When estrogen levels drop during perimenopause, menopause, and post menopause, those neurotransmitter systems get thrown off balance, leading to mood swings, irritability, anxiety, and even depression.

Cortisol Role in Mood Regulation

When you're under stress, your body releases a hormone called cortisol. It's part of your "fight or flight" system, designed to help you survive dangerous or high-pressure situations. In small doses, cortisol can help you stay alert and focused. But when it stays elevated too often (which happens more easily during menopause because of hormonal imbalances), it can cause irritability, anxiety, fatigue, sleep problems, and even brain fog.

Here's the kicker:

Estrogen normally helps regulate your body's stress response by keeping cortisol in check. But when estrogen levels drop during menopause, that natural buffering system weakens. As a result:

• You become more sensitive to stress.

• Minor frustrations feel overwhelming.

• Your ability to emotionally "bounce back" slows down.

This is why something as small as a snarky comment, a forgotten appointment, or a cluttered kitchen can feel like the last straw.

The Subcomponents of Emotional Stress: How Anxiety and Panic Take Hold

What makes up emotional stress? Let's break down the different components that shape it and explore how each one affects us in its own unique way. Stress is the body's reaction to a threat, while anxiety is the body's reaction to stress.

Anxiety

Anxiety is a natural response to stress or perceived danger. It's a feeling of unease, worry, or fear that can range from mild to intense. Anxiety often builds gradually and lingers—it's less like a storm and more like a heavy mist you walk through. An anxiety attack is usually a buildup of worries. For example, imagine you are driving and suddenly another car swerves into

your lane. In that moment, your heart races, your muscles tense, and your body goes into fight-or-flight mode, which is stress, your body's immediate reaction to a direct threat. Now, later that evening, even though you are safe at home, you find yourself replaying the situation in your mind. Your heart feels heavy, your chest is tight, and you cannot seem to relax. Even though the danger is long gone, your mind and body are reacting to the stress you experienced earlier. You are consumed with worrying, and you are worried about the outcome; this is what you call anxiety, your body's ongoing reaction to the memory of that stressful event. If you take it a step further and have an outburst, like snapping at someone nearby or breaking down into a deep, emotional cry, some people might say you are experiencing an anxiety attack.

Panic

Panic is an intense, overwhelming sense of fear or dread. A panic attack can be from an isolated situation that happened in your past. The panic attack comes out of nowhere, but sometimes it is something in the environment that triggers it, and at times it can be very subtle. It can be triggered by a real threat, imagined danger, or even sudden stress. Sometimes it's fleeting—like panicking when you lose your keys—or lingering, like a generalized sense of dread. A panic attack can come on suddenly and intensely, without warning, and often without a clear cause. It comes with a racing heart, difficulty breathing, trembling, dizziness, nausea, chest pain or tightness, sweating, and a feeling of losing control or impending doom, and fear of dying. It feels physical and severe.

The Overlap of Panic and Anxiety Attacks: Similar but Different

Now this may sound a bit confusing, so let me try to sum it up in simpler terms, but before I do that, the phrase anxiety attack is not an official medical term, but the phrase panic attack is an official medical term. In other words, you will not find the phrase anxiety attack in The DSM-5, which stands for the Diagnostic and Statistical Manual of Mental Disorders. It's the official handbook that mental health professionals in the U.S. (and many other countries) use to define, classify, and diagnose mental disorders.

Anxiety attacks often have a clear trigger; they usually come on gradually, there are more emotional symptoms, and they have a lingering duration. In a panic attack, the trigger may not always be so clear; it may come on suddenly, with more physical symptoms, and the duration is usually short.

Long-Term Effects

Menopause often magnifies emotional pressures, causing certain stressors to feel more overwhelming and harder to handle. Chronic stress can weaken the immune system, making the body more vulnerable to illness and disease. Ongoing stress and anxiety may also lead to persistently high blood pressure, increasing the risk of serious health problems over time. It disrupts healthy sleep patterns, leaving you exhausted and emotionally drained. For some, stress triggers emotional eating as a source of comfort, which can lead to unwanted weight gain and unhealthy habits that are difficult to break.

Taking Control of Your Emotions Before Stress Takes Control of You

Ladies, it is time to trade that runaway train for the guided Midnight Train to Georgia, where you can leave the drama behind and ride in the direction of your best, unbothered self. I struggled for a while to manage my emotions, but I learned that it is all about mindset and taking charge of what you can control and letting go of what you cannot control.

Releasing What We Can't Carry

Letting go isn't a sign of weakness—it's a radical act of trust. When we learn to release what we can't control, we give ourselves permission to stop carrying weight that was never ours to bear. Emotions like frustration, guilt, or anxiety often thrive in the gap between reality and expectation. When we consciously choose not to grip tightly to outcomes or others' reactions, we reclaim our peace. It's not about giving up—it's about giving space. In that space, clarity can breathe, resilience can grow, and emotional balance can return. We may not control the winds, but we can learn how to steady our sails.

Learning to Listen: The First Step to Healing Stress

What if, in the middle of our daily race, we actually honored the stop signs? Instead of blasting through them, what if we paused—just long enough to check in, breathe, and ask ourselves how we are doing? The moment we start to feel pressure creeping in could be our signal to slow down and recalibrate. Because sometimes, the most powerful move is not about pushing forward—it is pulling over for a moment of clarity.

When Emotions Rise, Respect Remains

While menopause brings undeniable emotional shifts, it's important to recognize that these changes do not excuse unkindness toward others. Hormonal fluctuations may heighten frustration, irritability, or even anger, but our words still carry weight and can leave a lasting impact. Conquering this begins with awareness — noticing the moments when emotions feel overwhelming. From there, practicing self-regulation strategies such as pausing before responding, journaling, breathing exercises, or stepping away from a heated moment allows us to respond with grace rather than react with harm. It's also about self-compassion: permitting ourselves to feel but choosing to express those feelings in ways that protect relationships. True strength in this journey is not found in denying our emotions, but in mastering how we express them.

3 Ways to Respond Instead of React

Pause Before Speaking: When emotions rise, give yourself a brief pause — even a few deep breaths. This small moment of space helps prevent words you might regret later. **Name the Feeling, Not the Blame:**

Instead of lashing out at someone, try saying what you're experiencing: "I'm feeling overwhelmed right now" rather than "You're making me upset." This shifts the focus from attacking to expressing. **Step Away to Reset:** If the moment feels too heated, it's okay to take a break. Step outside, journal your feelings, or practice grounding techniques. Returning with a calmer mind helps you respond with kindness.

Quieting the Noise Within

Stress doesn't announce itself with clarity; it creeps in quietly, disguising itself as restlessness, overwhelm, or even physical tension. In today's fast-paced world, it's easy to overlook the small signs until they've snowballed into emotional fatigue. That's why learning to recognize stress and respond with intention isn't just self-care—it's self-preservation. Before diving into practical strategies, let's pause and acknowledge the power of creating space: space to breathe, space to regroup, to gently reclaim control over what we feel and how we respond. The following tips are not quick fixes—they are invitations to soothe

the nervous system, foster resilience, and find your way back to equilibrium.

Breathing Exercises

One of the simplest yet most powerful tools we have to manage stress, tension, and anxiety is our breath. When we are overwhelmed, our breathing often becomes shallow and rapid, which keeps the body in a state of fight or flight. Breathing exercises work by slowing down the breath, signaling to the brain and nervous system that it is safe to relax. Deep, intentional breathing helps lower cortisol levels, ease muscle tension, and calm racing thoughts. It reconnects us to the present moment and pulls our focus away from anxious thinking. Regular breathing practices can reduce heart rate, improve sleep, and even stabilize blood pressure over time. It is not just about taking a deep breath; it is about creating a moment of stillness within chaos, giving your body permission to release what it is holding on to. In those few quiet moments, you take back control of your emotional and physical state, one steady breath at a time.

Focus on Belly Breathing. Place one hand on your chest and the other on your belly. Inhale slowly through your nose, letting your belly rise. Exhale gently through your mouth, feeling your belly fall. Try to keep your hand on your chest as still as possible. There was a moment for me when everything felt like too much—my thoughts racing, my body tense, my heart caught in the storm. But I remembered the breath. Slowly inhale, and the exhale... and with each cycle, a quiet return. It didn't fix the chaos outside, but it gave me space inside. Deep breathing became my anchor, reminding me I could choose presence over panic and peace over pressure.

Journaling

Journaling is one of the simplest, yet most powerful tools for managing emotional stress and restoring mental clarity. When you take the time to write out your thoughts, emotions, and frustrations, you give yourself a safe, judgment-free space to release what you might be holding inside. It allows you to process difficult feelings instead of bottling them up, which often leads to emotional overload. Beyond just venting, journaling helps you gain perspective by seeing your thoughts clearly on paper. Over time, it can reveal patterns in your emotional triggers, showing you what situations, people, or habits tend to disrupt your peace. This self-awareness is a powerful step toward healing because when you recognize what's affecting you, you're better equipped to manage it. Whether it's a few sentences at the end of the day or pages of raw emotion, journaling reconnects you with yourself in a way that calms the mind and soothes the heart. Write down every thought and feeling of frustration without holding back or overthinking it. Getting those emotions onto paper helps clear mental clutter and makes room for calm. I keep a few cue cards at my desk with simple reminders and affirmations. When I feel overwhelmed or frustrated, I glance at them, and it instantly grounds me, helping me avoid falling into an emotional spiral.

Laughter

Laughter is one of the most natural, overlooked forms of emotional medicine we have. It lightens the heart, soothes the mind, and instantly lifts the weight of heavy emotions. When you laugh even for a moment, your body releases feel-good chemicals like endorphins, which help reduce stress, ease physical tension, and improve your mood. But beyond the physical benefits, laughter heals the soul. It reminds you that joy still exists, even in the middle of life's toughest seasons. It reconnects you to the lighter, freer part of yourself that can get lost in the demands of daily life, especially during menopause, when emotions can feel unpredictable. Whether it comes from a funny memory, a comedy show, or a simple, silly moment with a loved one, laughter breaks through emotional heaviness and creates space for peace, gratitude, and perspective. It is a beautiful reminder that no matter what you are facing, light still lives within you. Laughter is a powerful tool.

Music Therapy

Music has a unique, almost magical way of reaching the parts of us that words alone cannot touch. It can calm an anxious mind, lift a weary spirit, and stir up joy even in life's hardest moments. Music therapy is more than just listening to a favorite song; it is intentionally using music to support emotional healing and well-being. Certain rhythms and melodies can ease tension, lower heart rate, and release emotional blockages you didn't even realize you were carrying. A slow, soothing tune can quiet racing thoughts, while an upbeat, joyful song can reignite hope and energy when you feel drained. Music connects you to memories, emotions, and parts of your soul that need care and attention. It becomes a gentle companion through grief, stress, and uncertainty — and a powerful tool for restoring peace, balance, and inner strength when words fall short.

Creative Outlets

Creative outlets (Hobbies) give your mind a healthy distraction and a positive focus when emotions start to take over. Creative outlets are powerful emotional release valves, offering a healthy way to process feelings that can be difficult to put into words. Whether it's painting, gardening, writing, dancing, crafting, or cooking, creative activities allow you to express what lives inside you without judgment or expectation. During times of stress, anxiety, or emotional heaviness, immersing yourself in something creative shifts your focus, quiets the mind, and reconnects you with the present moment. It's not about being perfect or producing something for others — it's about creating for yourself, allowing your heart and hands to work together to release what words sometimes cannot. Creative outlets nurture the soul, restore peace, and remind you that even in chaos, you have the power to build, shape, and bring beauty into your world. They are gentle, personal tools for healing, growth, and self-discovery.

Mindfulness & Meditation

Practicing mindfulness or guided meditation is one of the most effective ways to ease emotional overwhelm and reconnect with yourself. When stress builds and emotions feel out of control, the mind tends to race between past regrets and future worries, pulling you away from the present moment. Mindfulness gently brings your awareness back to the here and now, helping you recognize what you are feeling without judgment. Guided meditation can help slow your breathing, relax your muscles, and quiet the mental noise that fuels anxiety and tension. Even just 5 to 10 minutes a day of focus and intentional stillness can lower cortisol levels, improve clarity, and restore a sense of emotional calm. Over time, this simple practice can strengthen emotional resilience, reduce reactivity, and give you greater control over how you respond to daily stressors. It is a gentle, accessible tool that reminds you that you are in control of your peace.

Mindfulness & Meditation Practices to Calm Anxiety

Mindfulness Practices

1. Deep Breathing Breaks – Inhale for 4 counts, hold for 4, exhale for 6.

2. 5-Minute Body Scan – Notice where tension sits in your body and gently release it.

3. Mindful Walking – Focus on each step, your breath, and the feel of the ground beneath you.

4. Journaling Without Judgment -Write freely to release racing thoughts.

5. Mindful Eating – Slow down and savor each bite, noticing textures, flavors, and gratitude.

Meditation Practices

6. Guided Meditation – Use an app or YouTube for short, calming sessions. (Guided voice sessions → someone calmly talking you through breathing, relaxation, or visualization).

7. Loving-Kindness Meditation – Send compassion to yourself, loved ones, and even strangers.

8. Breath Awareness Meditation – Count inhales and exhales to anchor your mind.

9. Peaceful Visualization – Picture yourself in a calm, safe place (beach, garden, mountains).

10. Mantra Meditation – Repeat grounding words like *peace, calm*, or *I am safe.*

Connecting with Others

One of the most important yet often overlooked forms of emotional healing is connecting with others. Human connection is a natural remedy for isolation, anxiety, and emotional overwhelm. When you open up to someone you trust — whether it's a friend, family member, support group, or community of women walking a similar path — you remind yourself that you are not alone in what you are feeling. Sharing your experiences, your highs and lows, and simply being heard can lighten the emotional load you carry. It offers validation, comfort, and perspective in moments when you feel unseen or misunderstood, especially during menopause, when emotional changes can feel isolating. Connecting with others can restore hope, bring laughter back into your life, and create a circle of encouragement that reminds you of your strength. Emotional wellness often begins with a simple conversation and the courage to reach out.

Setting Boundaries

Setting boundaries is an essential act of self-care, especially during emotionally demanding seasons like menopause. It means recognizing your limits and permitting yourself to protect your time, energy, and emotional space. So often, women are conditioned to pour into everyone else while silently neglecting their own needs. But without clear boundaries, stress, anxiety, and emotional burnout quickly follow. Saying no to unnecessary obligations, limiting time with people who drain you, and prioritizing your own well-being is not selfish — it's necessary. Boundaries create space for you to breathe, heal, and focus on what truly matters to you. They remind you that your needs, peace, and emotional health deserve to come first sometimes. The more you practice honoring those boundaries, the stronger, more balanced, and emotionally grounded you become. Setting boundaries was one of my biggest challenges, but over time, I learned to replace many of my 'yeses' with more 'no's to protect my well-being.

Prioritizing Sleep

Prioritizing quality sleep is essential for managing stress and maintaining emotional balance, especially during menopause when sleep disruptions are common. Poor sleep doesn't just leave you tired; it amplifies stress hormones and heightens emotional sensitivity, making it harder to cope with daily challenges. Establishing a healthy bedtime routine can

make a significant difference. This might include
limiting screen time before bed, as the blue light from
devices interferes with your body's natural sleep
signals. Incorporating relaxation practices like gentle
stretching, deep breathing, or listening to calming
music can prepare your mind and body for restful
sleep. By protecting your sleep, you give yourself a
powerful foundation to face the next day with greater
resilience, clarity, and calm.

Embracing your emotional journey through menopause

Embracing your emotional journey through
menopause means honoring every feeling that arises,
even the difficult ones. It's about recognizing that
your emotions are not a sign of weakness, but rather a
reflection of the profound changes happening within
you—physically, mentally, and spiritually. This
journey invites you to slow down, listen deeply to
yourself, and offer compassion where before there
may have been judgment or frustration. When you
accept your emotions as valid and necessary, you
reclaim your power to heal and grow. Each emotional

wave and moment of vulnerability becomes a doorway to greater resilience and a new narrative for this transformative chapter.

As you step into this next chapter of your life, you can look forward to a season of renewed clarity, purpose, and freedom. Menopause is not an ending—it is a powerful beginning that invites you to redefine what vitality and joy mean on your own terms. This phase offers the chance to shed old expectations and embrace your authentic self with confidence and grace. You'll discover deeper self-awareness, stronger intuition, and a richer connection to your body and spirit. With the tools, support, and resilience you're cultivating now, you're prepared to create a life that reflects your true values and desires—one filled with balance, peace, and meaningful growth. The journey ahead holds endless possibilities for transformation, empowerment, and radiant well-being.

The Truth About Setbacks and Emotional Growth

I want to be clear from the start: this book is not a cure-all. Life isn't perfect, and none of us are. There will be times when setbacks happen, and that's completely normal. My goal is not to promise that reading these pages will magically erase every emotional struggle. What I do hope is that this book can inspire and guide you. You may already know some of these strategies I share, and just reading about them is not enough. The real value comes when you allow these ideas to minister to your heart and mind and then take action to apply them in your life. That is when you begin to handle your emotions in healthier, more balanced ways.

I also want to be honest about myself: I don't have it all together, and I still experience setbacks. The difference now is that I've learned to navigate my emotions without letting them drain me. That is what I hope to share with you — not perfection, but tools, perspective, and encouragement so you can manage your feelings with more ease and confidence.

Steering Your Emotional Journey

Understanding your emotional landscape means you are no longer at the mercy of your feelings—you become the conscious guide steering through the highs and lows with grace and courage. Resilience is not about avoiding pain or discomfort; it's about showing up for yourself fully, even when the path feels uncertain. You carry within you a wellspring of strength, wisdom, and grace that menopause only begins to uncover. By embracing your emotional journey, you are stepping into a new chapter of life marked by self-awareness, authenticity, and renewed confidence. This is your time to rise, to thrive, and to embody the powerful woman you truly are

Conclusion

Managing stress and emotions is not just about feeling better in the moment — it's about reclaiming control over your life and health during a time when your body and mind face unique challenges. Menopause can amplify emotional ups and downs, making everyday stressors feel overwhelming. Techniques like breathing exercises, mindfulness, journaling, and creative outlets provide practical, accessible ways to calm the mind, process difficult feelings, and restore balance. They help interrupt the cycle of anxiety and tension, giving you tools to respond rather than react to emotional triggers.

Beyond immediate relief, these practices support long-term well-being by strengthening emotional resilience, improving sleep, and reducing the physical toll of chronic stress. Connecting with others and setting healthy boundaries protects your energy and fosters a sense of belonging and safety. Together, these strategies create a holistic approach to emotional health that empowers you to face menopause not just with survival in mind, but with confidence, strength, and renewed joy. Remember, setbacks are a natural part of life, and no one navigates this journey perfectly. With the right knowledge, tools, and resources, you can move through challenges with resilience, grace, and confidence. That's the heart of Beyond the Footprints of Menopause—each footprint that honors not perfection but progress, resilience, and the courage to keep moving forward.

Affirmation: *"I welcome each emotional wave with compassion and courage. What I feel is valid, what I release is healing, and what I become is powerful."*

CHAPTER 3
The Physical Weight We Carry

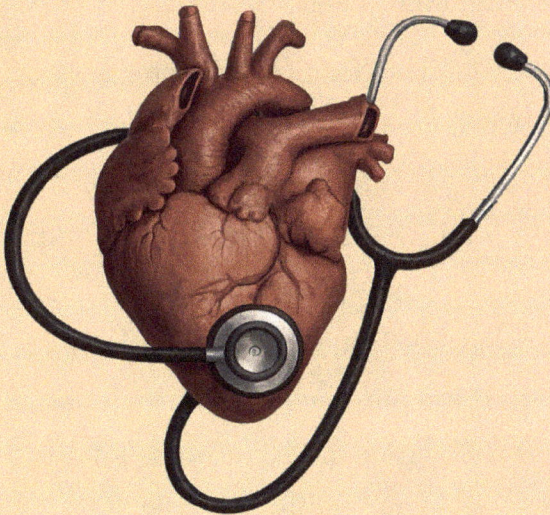

3 The Other Half of the Story: The Physical Weight We Carry

The journey doesn't stop at the emotional challenges; we also face physical challenges. Menopause is not just a change in cycles; it's a stage where women become significantly more vulnerable to chronic conditions if early signs are ignored. The Hormone Transition—when will it relent? How much strain can our bodies and minds bear?

While society tends to focus heavily on the emotional aspects — which are undeniably important — the physical realities we face are just as significant. The truth is, our bodies endure constant shifts and challenges during this season of life, and physical experiences deserve just as much attention and compassion. It is a partnership. If our minds are not functioning well, how can we truly care for our bodies? And when our bodies are struggling, it becomes even harder to care for our mental and emotional well-being. The two are deeply connected — one affects the other, and both deserve our attention.

At this point, you might wonder: What can you do when your mind and body feel out of sync? The truth is, it's not about fixing everything at once. It's about recognizing where you are, giving yourself grace, and taking small, intentional steps. When both your mental and physical health are struggling, the first step is awareness—acknowledging how you are feeling without judgment. From there, it's about choosing one small thing you can do to nurture either your body or your mind, because even the smallest act of care in one area can begin to lift the other. Healing is not instant, but it is possible when we stop chasing perfection and start embracing progress.

Unfortunately, this was my story. I'm not sure where this mindset originated, but I grew up thinking that I had to do everything perfectly. My husband, at one time, stated that I had obsessive-compulsive behavior. Even today, I am still unsure whether he was joking or serious. This doesn't mean I was perfect — far from it. What I struggled with was perfectionism, the constant drive to do everything flawlessly. It may sound admirable, but in reality, perfectionism can fuel stress, self-criticism, and eventually burnout. As I entered my menopause phase, the pressure to be perfect only grew heavier, and the toll it took on me became even worse. I came to realize that unless I let go of the constant need to be perfect and do everything right, I was headed straight for burnout—and possibly a hospital bed.

The Silent Whispers

We've all been there—going to the doctor with symptoms and hearing, yet again, that it's probably just stress. It can be frustrating, and it's totally okay to get a second opinion—you deserve that. However, if the tests continue to come back clear, perhaps it's time to seriously consider how much stress is affecting your health. Often, it's our loved ones, family, or friends who notice the stress we're under before we recognize it ourselves. Often, we find ourselves in denial about the extent of the stress we're carrying. There is research out there that suggests stress can cause a multitude of physical ailments. It's easy to dismiss the subtle whispers our body sends—the lingering fatigue, the persistent ache, the shift in mood or sleep—because life demands so much of us. We push through, adapt, normalize the discomfort, and tell ourselves it's just aging or stress. But those signs aren't meant to be silenced; they're signals. Our body doesn't speak in words—it speaks in symptoms. When something is off, it doesn't betray us; it alerts us. Ignoring those messages doesn't make them go away—it just delays the opportunity to heal.

Your Body Is Not the Enemy: Partnering with Your Body Through Menopause and Beyond

The truth is that our body is on our side. It's not trying to hold us back—it's trying to protect us, redirect us, sometimes even slow us down for our own good. When we begin to tune in instead of tuning out, we uncover a whole new level of partnership with ourselves. That's when real transformation begins, not by pushing harder, but by listening deeper. The journey through menopause, or any major health transition, becomes a doorway—not to disconnection, but to reconnection. And your body? It's not the enemy. It's the guide. Stress isn't just something we feel in our minds. It leaves its mark on the body as well. When we carry stress day after day, our bodies take notice, and over time, the body starts to respond in ways we can't ignore. Headaches, weight gain, insomnia, high blood pressure, and digestive issues are just a few of the warning signs. Chronic stress can lead to serious health problems like heart disease, stroke, autoimmune disorders, and even mental health challenges like anxiety and depression. The body keeps score of every sleepless night, every anxious thought, and every unresolved emotion. That's why it's so important to listen, to pay attention to what your body is trying to tell you, and to take action before those stress signals turn into something far more dangerous. The first step, of course, is to identify what's causing stress. Only then can we begin to manage the physical symptoms that tag along with it. Many health issues linked to stress can be brought under control once we pinpoint the source. Physical conditions such as hypertension, palpitations, stomach issues, and others can be managed.

Healing From the Inside Out

I had all of these symptoms during my menopause phase, and then some. In the beginning, I did not want to admit that stress could be the cause of my symptoms. I found myself in the doctor's office time and time again, undergoing every test imaginable—CAT scans, X-rays, ultrasounds—you name it. I became the queen of medical testing, hoping someone could finally tell me what was wrong. I finally realized that maybe, just maybe, I need to control my stress level. When I began to discover the source of my stress level, I began to learn how to control my high blood pressure, my palpitations, and my stomach issues. It was a turning point for me. The moment I shifted from searching for answers outside of myself to tuning in and asking, What is my body trying to tell me? I realized that no machine could scan what I was carrying emotionally: the weight of constant pressure, unspoken expectations, and the internalized belief that I just had to keep going. Once I began managing the stress—and truly exploring where it was coming from—my body started to respond. It didn't need another test; it needed space and permission to heal. That is when I began creating my path to wellness— one grounded in awareness rather than avoidance. Healing from the inside out means giving your body what it needs to restore balance in its natural systems — digestion, detoxification, immunity, and the nervous system— so they can do what they were designed to do: protect, repair, and restore. When these systems are nurtured through proper nutrition, regular movement, emotional release, and restful sleep, chronic conditions become less likely to develop.

Healing from the inside out involves building resilience: nourishing the body with whole foods, reducing toxic load, managing stress, and creating space for joy. It's not about perfection; it's about creating a lifestyle that supports your internal environment, promoting longevity and vitality. When a woman commits to understanding and honoring what her body is truly asking for, she no longer feels like she's fighting it — she feels like she's partnering with it. And that's where prevention becomes power.

Before the Prescription

Sometimes, we believe that taking medication for every ailment is the ultimate solution. And let me be clear, I am not saying you should avoid the medications your doctor prescribed. There are certain conditions where medication is necessary for your body to heal and function properly. If you have high blood pressure, and taking the medications is necessary, take your medication as prescribed by your doctor. If your blood sugar is dangerously high and your doctor says it's time for medication, listen to your physician. Diabetes can be a very nasty disease that causes all types of problems. As a Registered Nurse and having worked at the bedside for over 20 years, I watched patients lose their limbs due to diabetes. Diabetes is nothing to take lightly. Does this mean you'll need to stay on these medications for the rest of your life? For some, no, but you should never stop taking your medications without creating a plan with your doctor. In certain cases, people who made lifestyle changes through nutrition and stress management were able to reduce or even come off their medications. However, this should always be a decision made in partnership with your physician. What I am talking about are those moments when you visit your doctor, and your numbers are creeping up — your blood pressure is a little high, or your labs are borderline — and instead of jumping straight to medication at that particular time, your doctor advises you to make lifestyle changes first: lose some weight, lower your salt and fat intake, and get more rest. Too often, we brush it off and don't take it seriously enough until it reaches a point where medication becomes the only option. The truth is, when you're overwhelmed with stress, it can be incredibly difficult to take control of your health. But ignoring those early interventions only pushes you closer to needing medications you might have been able to avoid. The key is stepping in early—tuning in to your body's signals and taking action now—so you stay in control of your health, not the other way around. Manage your blood pressure before it manages you, and you'll avoid consequences that never have to happen. Again, listen to the body's early silent whispers before they become screams.

True healing begins within — not just in the absence of disease, but in the presence of balance. When we talk about preventing chronic illness, it's not about waiting for a diagnosis and then reacting—it's about cultivating internal harmony now. That harmony can be disrupted long before symptoms appear, as inflammation, blood sugar imbalances, and gut disruptions often build up slowly over years of stress, nutrient depletion, poor sleep, and emotional overload.

When Stress Hits the Heart: Protecting Your Most Vital Organ

Heart disease is the number one killer in women. The sad part about it is that less than half of the women recognize heart disease as the greatest threat to their health. In my last years as a bedside nurse, my specialty was cardiac care, and even today, it is still a passion of mine. As a Case Manager specializing in disease management, I spent years coaching both men and women on heart health. Today, as a health coach, my passion lies in guiding women to care for their whole selves in their menopausal years and not just managing the symptoms of menopause. I stress the importance of caring for your heart because a healthy heart is the foundation of your overall well-being.

When you are under stress, your body triggers a "fight or flight" response. This causes the brain to release stress hormones like adrenaline and cortisol, which immediately increase the heart rate, raise blood pressure, and make your heart work harder than usual. Over time, if stress becomes chronic, this constant strain can damage the heart and blood vessels. Chronic stress can contribute to high blood pressure (hypertension), irregular heart rhythms (like palpitations), an increased risk of heart attack or stroke, plaque buildup in the arteries that can cause blockages, and elevated cholesterol levels can contribute to these problems. Protecting the heart during high-stress seasons means shifting from reacting to prevention. It's about calming your nervous system through intentional rest, mindful breathing, gentle movement, and genuine connection — not only with others, but with your own body's wisdom. Prioritizing joy, setting boundaries, and addressing unresolved emotions are not luxuries — they're heart health strategies. True transformation begins when we recognize the heart not just as a muscle, but as the center of our emotional and physical well-being.

Don't Wait for a Diagnosis: Menopause Is Your Window to Take Control

Neglecting your health during menopause can quietly set the stage for long-term consequences that are far more difficult to reverse later. As hormones shift, a woman's risk for serious conditions like osteoporosis, heart disease, high blood pressure, insulin resistance, and cognitive decline can increase, but often without dramatic warning signs. What starts as fatigue, weight gain, or irregular sleep can escalate into chronic ailments that affect every area of life. Ignoring your body's cues during this pivotal phase doesn't just delay healing; it allows imbalance to take root. Prioritizing your health now is not just self-care; it's disease prevention, and it's one of the most powerful gifts you can give your future self. When you pause and become aware of its presence, you give yourself the power to do something about it. You are now in control.

When the Body Speaks: Turning Stress Signals into Self-Care

The sooner you acknowledge your body's subtle stress signals, the sooner you can intervene—soothing your nervous system, clearing your mind, and preventing those silent health risks from taking root. Awareness is your first line of defense. Intentional action is your power move. But let's be honest—we all know why we brush off those early signs. Our bodies whisper, "slow down," but we've been conditioned to speed up. In a world that praises hustle and treats exhaustion like a badge of honor, pausing feels like failure. Still, your body is not the enemy—it's your most loyal ally. Under pressure, it doesn't betray you. It tries to protect you. So, ask yourself: Is the finish line worth racing toward if you arrive burned out and broken? You may not control the pace of the world, but you do control the rhythm of your own life. Unaddressed emotions don't just disappear; they can often transform into physical symptoms that affect your well-being.

This chapter was not written to teach you how to treat heart disease, high blood pressure, or any other physical conditions. My goal here is simple and urgent: to remind you that small, intentional changes made today can transform your well-being for years to come. Stress is not just emotional—it's physiological. It can place real physical strain on the body, draining energy, disrupting balance, and impacting your overall well-being.

The Path Forward: Trusting Your Signals to Protect Your Health

You have more influence than you've been told. You can interrupt the cycle. You can choose to listen now, before your body has to shout to get your attention. Before we go any further, let's talk about trusting yourself—and learning to listen to what your symptoms are telling you. That trust begins the moment you pause, notice, and say, I matter enough to respond to what I feel. The path to lasting health isn't paved with guesswork — it's shaped by tuning into the body's signals and honoring what they're trying to communicate. So often, women are taught to dismiss discomfort, power through fatigue, or silence their symptoms with quick fixes. Our bodies are intelligent — sending us whispers long before they escalate into cries for help. Whether it's persistent bloating, brain fog, mood swings, or joint pain, each cue is an invitation to pause, evaluate, and take action. When we begin to trust those signals instead of overriding them, we shift from reactive care to preventative empowerment. Especially during menopause, listening to the body becomes more than just a wellness practice — it becomes a lifeline. Hormonal changes can mask or magnify symptoms, making it all the more critical to stay attuned. By developing a deeper awareness of what feels balanced versus what feels off, we can intervene earlier, protect our long-term health, and build resilience from the inside out. The path forward is not about perfection — it's about partnership. With your body, with your intuition, and with the tools that help you thrive.

Now That You're Listening, It's Time to Lead Yourself

With that awareness comes power. You can begin designing a lifestyle that supports healing rather than one that simply gets you through the day. This might mean setting boundaries that protect your peace, rebalancing your schedule to include joy and rest, or seeking out guidance from practitioners who see you as a whole person. Listening to the whispers was step one — but responding to them with courage and consistency is the next step. That's how you reclaim your health, rhythm, and voice. This is where transformation begins. Now that you have finally paused and begun to tune into the whispers of your body, the next step is to respond with intention. That means taking action that aligns with what your body is asking for — not rushing to "fix" everything, but creating space to nourish, restore, and recalibrate. Maybe it looks like adjusting your nutrition to calm inflammation, prioritizing sleep, journaling to release buried emotions, or starting a gentle movement practice that feels energizing instead of exhausting.

This is the moment to shift from ignoring those whispers to exploring root causes — because now, you are not ignoring the signs, you are honoring them.

Once a woman has heard her body's whispers and chooses to respond, the next step is equipping herself with practical strategies to promote physical healing, which might include targeted lab work to check hormone levels, inflammation markers, or nutrient deficiencies — not to chase a diagnosis, but to uncover imbalances that can be restored. From there, tools like an anti-inflammatory nutrition plan, strength training, pelvic floor exercises, and breathwork can help support hormone health, gut integrity, and nervous system regulation. These aren't one-size-fits-all solutions — they're personalized steps, chosen based on how your body is showing up.

Equally important is having a trusted team and reliable resources. A functional medicine practitioner, a women's health coach, or even a menopause literate therapist who can help guide the journey and tailor support. Tools like symptom trackers, guided meditation, and books alike can start you on your way

as well. This is about creating a support system —
body, mind, and community — so you don't have to
navigate healing alone. You are not waiting for
someone else to fix you anymore; you are actively
participating in your own transformation.

Conclusion

As estrogen levels drop in menopause, your risk for
serious health issues rises, highlighting the need to
listen to your body and act proactively. This chapter
was not just about recognizing your symptoms — it
was about reclaiming your role as the most powerful
advocate for your own well-being. When you begin to
trust your body's signals, respond with intention, and
gather the tools to support your unique journey, you
move from not just surviving the menopausal
transition but to actively shaping it. You're no longer
waiting for someone to permit you to heal; you're
giving it to yourself. Your body is sending you
messages—listen closely, act decisively, and take back
control before the condition takes control of you.
Ignoring your physical symptoms allows them to write
your story; paying attention gives you the pen. Don't

wait for a crisis to force action—honor your body today, because prevention is the ultimate power. Your health is not something to gamble with. Recognize the signals, respond with intention, and reclaim your vitality. Every symptom is an invitation to act. Step forward now, before your body dictates the terms.

You are not broken. Your body is not your enemy. This season, as complex and challenging as it may be, can also become the turning point — the moment you rise into a more present, powerful, and whole version of yourself. Each choice you make to honor your body is a footprint toward healing: steady, intentional, and entirely your own.

Affirmation: *"I honor the signals my body sends and meet them with grace. Each moment of awareness is a step toward balance, and each act of care is a promise I keep to myself. I am not behind—I am becoming. And in this becoming, I trust my body to lead the way, and I trust myself to follow."*

CHAPTER 4
A SPIRITUAL JOURNEY

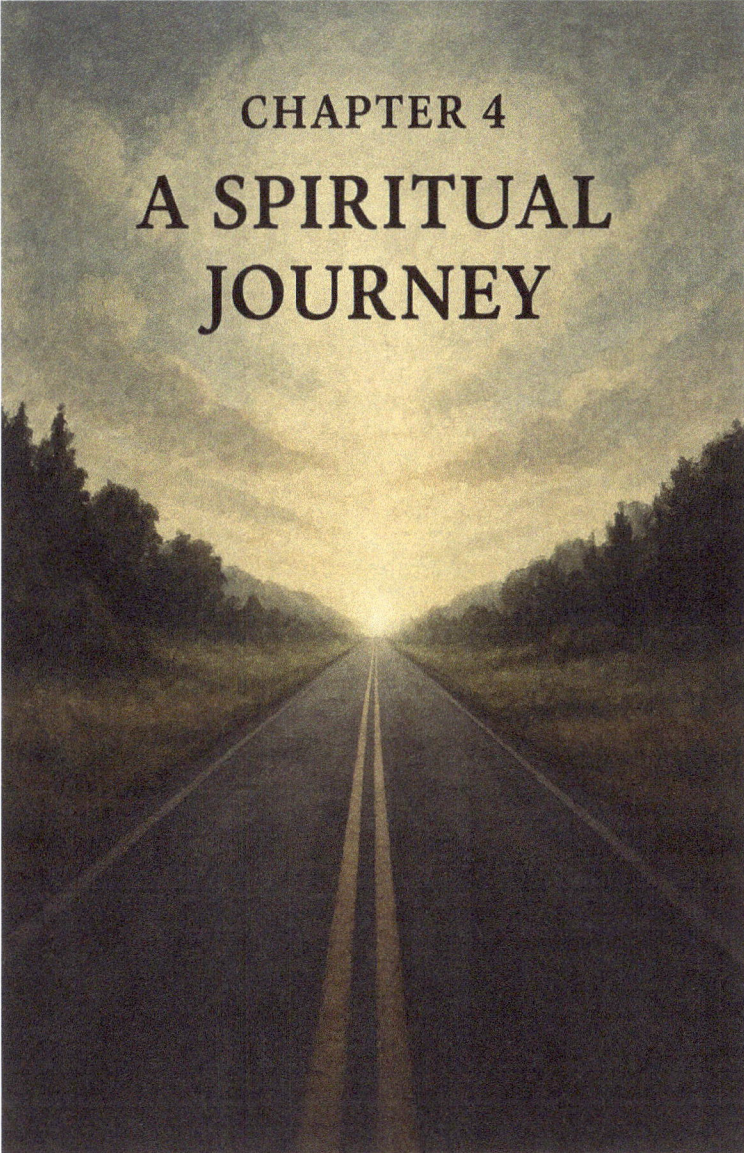

4 A Spiritual Journey: Trusting God's Guidance Through the Seasons of Change

When we go through menopause, many of us experience moments that feel heavier than we ever expected. The emotional highs and lows, the sleepless nights, the unexpected shifts in our bodies and minds can pull us into some very dark, isolating places. During these times, it's not uncommon for our faith to waver. What once felt steady and unshakable can suddenly feel distant or uncertain. I've had seasons where my connection to God felt strong and comforting, and other times when I questioned everything, wondering if he was still listening. It is important to acknowledge that this is a normal part of both the human and spiritual experience. Faith doesn't always feel steady — some days it stands firm, and other days it wavers, especially in the face of life-changing transitions like menopause. In those darker moments, even a small spark of faith — a whispered prayer, a quiet moment of reflection, or simply the act of getting out of bed and trying again — can be enough to keep moving forward. In this chapter, I will talk openly about the challenges of faith, and how reconnecting with your beliefs — whatever they look like for you — can become a powerful source of strength, healing, and hope during times of change.

I'm not sure what your personal beliefs are, what faith you follow, or where you are on your spiritual path right now — and that's okay. We all come to this part of our journey from different places. In this chapter, I want to be transparent with you. For me, it's been my relationship with God that has held me together in the most difficult moments of my life, especially during the emotional twists and turns that happen during my menopause journey. My faith has been a steady anchor when everything else felt uncertain. I'll be sharing how leaning on God's guidance, grace, and strength helped me navigate this season and how reconnecting with the spiritual part — whatever that looks like for you — can be a powerful part of healing, growth, and rediscovery.

Grace in the Gaps: It's the Return That Matters

Some days, I would wake up not feeling so great and would get on my knees and pray, asking God to get me through the day as I travel through this menopause journey. There would be other days, I didn't pray or ask for guidance, and I would beat myself up because I hadn't prayed on that certain day. But here's what I've learned: you don't have to feel bad when you miss a day of prayer. God's love isn't measured by our perfect consistency — it's about a relationship, not a routine. Grace meets us where we are, even in our silence. Whether you pray every morning or go days without a word, you are still held, still seen, and still deeply loved. What matters most is the return — the willingness to reconnect, even after the quiet.

Remembering While Hurting

We are emotional, thinking beings, and our minds naturally question and wrestle with things we can't fully control or predict. In moments of pain, loss, or uncertainty — especially during difficult seasons like illness or personal crises — our emotional distress can cloud the memory of past blessings. The immediate weight of suffering often feels heavier than the memory of past miracles.

Even when God has shown up for us before, a new trial can feel newly unbearable. It's like walking through a storm you've never weathered, even though you survived other storms before. The fear of what if this time is different, or what if he doesn't come through this time, can creep in because each struggle brings its own unique emotional and spiritual challenges.

Spiritual Fatigue Is Real

Constant battles — whether physical, emotional, or spiritual — wear people down. Even the strongest believer can get spiritually exhausted. Just as physical exhaustion weakens the body, spiritual fatigue can dull our sense of hope and connection, making it harder to feel God's presence or recall His track record in our lives.

The Silent Times Test Us the Most

There are moments when God seems silent. Even if we have experienced answered prayers before, seasons of silence can feel like abandonment, leading to doubts like "Where is He now?" or "Why does His voice seem silent right now?" Those silent seasons challenge our faith, yet even in the discomfort, God is shaping us—though doubts may try to surface.

Faith Is Not a Transaction

Faith is not a transaction where every prayer gets an immediate yes. It's a relationship — and like any relationship, there are high points, misunderstandings, questions, and periods of distance. The beauty of faith is not in never doubting, but in choosing to return even after we've questioned.

We often think that strong faith means having unshakable certainty, but real faith makes room for the wrestle. It allows us to bring our confusion, our disappointment, even our silence — and know we are still held. There's no punishment for being human. God isn't keeping a scorecard of our good days versus our doubtful ones. What matters is that we come back, again and again. We should stay open to reconnecting, even when we don't feel spiritual or strong.

Having The Faith of A Mustard Seed

In short, people's faith wavers because we are human. We hurt, we fear, we get tired. In those vulnerable places, our faith can shrink, no matter how many past prayers were answered. The incredible thing, though, is that even a flicker of faith, however small, still counts. The bible talks about having the faith of a mustard seed, which means even a little faith, God will still hear you and carry you from the heart of the storm into His peace. Often, it's in those moments of wavering that our faith deepens because we learn to trust not just in what God has done before, but in who he is, even when we don't feel it.

God Walks With You Through the Storm

God doesn't always prevent storms from coming into our lives. The hard seasons, the heartaches, the unexpected changes — they still arrive, whether we're ready or not. But what he promises is to walk through these storms with us. It is in those turbulent moments when the wind is howling, and the weight feels unbearable, that prayer becomes more than a routine; it becomes a lifeline commitment. Prayer isn't always about asking God to take the storm away, but about asking for the strength to endure it, the peace to quiet our anxious hearts, and the wisdom to trust that there's purpose even in the struggle. I have learned that sometimes God calms the storm around me, and other times, he calms the storm within me. Either way, his presence is the constant that steadies my spirit when everything else feels unsteady. If you find yourself in a storm right now, know that you don't have to face it alone. Prayer can become your anchor, grounding you in hope when the world feels out of control. Again, God does hear and answer prayers, but his answers may come in different ways (yes, no, or wait) and in his timing, not always yours.

I will never forget those devastating days during the COVID pandemic, when so many of us experienced heartbreaking losses of loved ones, friends, church members, family members, including husbands, wives, and children who were taken far too soon. As I was navigating changes and challenges in my menopause journey, another challenge came and knocked me down again. My son caught a very bad case of COVID. My son spent 30 days in the hospital, which included 17 days in the intensive care unit. This was one of the darkest chapters in both my husband's life and mine. My son's physical condition declined quickly. His oxygen levels were not stable, so he was put on a non-invasive ventilator. Both of his lungs partially collapsed, and bilateral chest tubes were placed. It is possible to be uncertain about what God will do, while still trusting who God is. Trust in God doesn't always mean being certain about the specific results — it means resting in His goodness and plan even when the result is unknown. The hospital staff actually let me stay with my son, and I spent every night in the hospital, in the intensive care unit at his bedside. Even though I was a Registered Nurse, I felt helpless at times, but I knew I had to stay strong for my son. He would look over at me with labored breathing—42 to 52 breaths per minute—and oxygen levels only in the 80's. He didn't say anything, but his eyes asked the question: Mommy, am I going to make it? By the grace of God and through prayer day in and day out, from everyone, which included all of his friends, family members, pastors, even my pastor, he made it through. My son stated he could feel the spirit of prayers all around him. He even told his friends on social media, the night the chest tubes were being inserted, "COVID, don't have me." God has me." That night, my faith became even stronger. God heard our prayers. He healed my son. Again, GOD does not always prevent the storms, but he helps you get through them. Did my son have a long recovery phase after he was discharged from the hospital? Yes, he did. Is he 100% today? No, he is not, but God kept him here with our prayers. He can function in life with minor health challenges.

Even if you are not consistent with prayer, never stop praying, never give up on God, because he is a forgiving God and he will never give up on you. It always reminds me that I don't have to face anything alone, and no matter how stormy life gets, God's presence is always there, steady, faithful, and waiting for me to reach out.

Staying Connected to God and His Word

"Over the years, I've come to understand that my connection with God does not have to be complicated or formal. It's about a relationship, not a ritual. For me, staying connected to God isn't about perfection or long, rehearsed prayers; Again, it's about a relationship. I've learned that the more I invite him into the small, ordinary moments of my day, the stronger my connection with him becomes. I start my mornings with quiet time, even if it's just five minutes, thanking him for another day and asking for guidance, wisdom, and peace to carry me through whatever's ahead. I've made it a habit to talk to God throughout the day, like I would a trusted friend. Some days, it's through journaling a simple prayer or reading a few verses of a scripture from the Bible. I also take some of my favorite scriptures and place them in my work area, and I have a necklace made with a scripture on it that I wear every day. Other times, it's just sitting in silence, listening to that still, small voice that reminds me I'm never alone. Then there is the prayer. As I stated before, even on days when I fell short in prayer, I never stopped turning to God and sharing my heart with Him. Keeping God at the center of my life means including him in the highs and the lows, not just when moments are going right and not just when moments are going wrong. It's in those little conversations I have with him throughout the day — thanking him for a beautiful sunset, asking for patience in a stressful moment, or leaning on his strength when my emotions feel overwhelming. It's not about how much time you spend or how eloquent your words are; it's about intention, presence, and letting God weave himself into the fabric of your daily life. The more we nurture that connection, the more peace, clarity, and strength we find, even in life's hardest seasons. Keep praying, keep believing, and keep walking in faith, even when it feels quiet. Some of our greatest spiritual growth happens in the waiting. I can say without a doubt, it truly happened to me.

Healing Starts Here: Anchoring Your Menopause Journey in Faith and Prayer

So, where do you begin? If you're feeling lost, weary, or like you're running on empty, the first step is not to fix everything—it's simply to pause. Create a quiet space, whether it's early morning or before bed, even for just a few minutes a day, where you can be still with your thoughts and invite God's presence into the moment. Be honest—tell him how you feel. You don't have to have the perfect words. Honest Prayer: Begin

94

with a real, unfiltered conversation. If you're frustrated, weary, or lost, speak it. Prayer isn't about perfection—it's about presence. Even a whisper of "Lord, help me" is powerful. Healing begins with real talk and raw truth between you and your creator. Allow prayer to become your anchor. This is not about performance—it is about a connection.

From there, open your Bible and sit with verses that remind you of his strength when yours feels gone. Let the words wash over you, letting His promises sink deep into your heart. Meditate on His faithfulness and let His presence fill the spaces where worry or fear may linger. Allow yourself to rest in the assurance that He is with you, carrying you through every challenge. Allow the stories and scriptures to wash over you, filling your heart with peace and strength. Let them remind you of hope, courage, and God's unwavering presence. Let these words become anchors, keeping your faith steady even in the midst of challenges.

Verses of Peace for the Journey

You might find a verse below that speaks to your heart. Add it to your favorite verses and carry it with you as a quiet reminder of His love. Some of my favorites are:

Psalm 34:17 (NIV) "The righteous cry out, and the Lord hears them; he delivers them from all their troubles."

Isaiah 40:31 (NIV) "But those who hope in the Lord will renew their strength. They will soar on wings like eagles; they will run and not grow weary; they will walk and not be faint."

Proverbs 3:6 (NIV) "Trust in the Lord with all your heart and lean not on your own understanding; in all your ways submit to him, and he will make your paths straight."

Write it down. Reflect on it. Speak it aloud.

Simple Spiritual Habits That Keep the Healing Going

1. Healing Journal: Keep a notebook by your side. Let it hold your prayers, questions, and breakthroughs. Start journaling your thoughts, your prayers, and the

whispers of reassurance He sends your way. What brings you peace? What needs to be let go of? Write freely, without judgment, allowing your heart to pour out all that is heavy or joyful. Record the moments you feel His presence, the small victories, and the lessons learned in quiet reflection. Over time, your journal becomes a map of His faithfulness, a reminder of how far you've come, and a testament to the ways He meets you even in the smallest detail. Journaling invites clarity and reveals what your spirit already knows.

2. Worship & Reflection Playlist: Create a playlist that soothes and lifts your soul. Include worship songs, instrumentals, or even calming affirmations. Music is medicine for the heart—it stirs joy, stillness, and release. Music heals my soul. When I was going through the worst of my emotional menopause journey some years ago, I started to dance to spiritual music that filled the hole in my soul. This led me to start a dance ministry called My Joy, a reflection of the deep joy I feel when dancing for Jesus. To this day, I continue to dance at churches and other events.

3. Community & Support: Healing doesn't happen in isolation. Connect with a sister circle, a prayer group, or a trusted coach. Invite safe conversations and mutual encouragement into your life.

These simple rhythms are not just routines—they're lifelines. Little by little, this spiritual grounding becomes the soil where emotional and physical healing can take root and grow. With each intentional moment, whether prayer, meditation, or quiet reflection, you nurture your spirit and strengthen your resilience. Over time, these small practices shape your perspective, bringing clarity, peace, and a deeper sense of connection to God. What may start as a simple habit can blossom into a steady source of hope, sustaining you through life's storms and joys alike.

Forgiving Yourself and Others as a Spiritual Release

Menopause and midlife often stir up more than just physical changes. This season of life has a way of bringing old memories, regrets, and unresolved emotions to the surface. Past betrayals, disappointments, and mistakes we thought we had buried long ago can suddenly feel fresh again. Many women carry silent burdens — resentment toward others who hurt them, guilt over things they wish they had done differently, or bitterness about unfair circumstances. What I have come to realize is that holding onto those wounds does not punish the people who caused them; it only keeps us spiritually bound to negative emotions. Unforgiveness acts like a weight on your spirit, clouding your peace and blocking your connection with God. It robs you of the freedom he wants you to experience.

Forgiveness is not about forgetting what happened or pretending it didn't hurt. It's about choosing to release the hold that those emotions have on your heart. It is not excusing someone's behavior but rather deciding that their actions no longer have the power to steal your joy and peace. Sometimes, the hardest person to forgive is yourself. We all carry things we wish we could undo — words we said in anger, seasons where we were not the person we wanted to be, choices we regret, but God's grace isn't partial or limited. The same forgiveness he offers others; he offers to you. When you finally decide to lay those burdens down and forgive others and yourself, you'll find a peace you did not realize you were missing. It's in that spiritual release that you make room for joy, healing, and a deeper relationship with God.

Reflection Prompt

Take a quiet moment to reflect: Is there someone you need to forgive, including yourself? Write down their names, situations, or even emotions you have been carrying. Then, ask God to help you release them one by one. You don't have to have all the answers today, but you can start the process of letting go.

Embracing my faith didn't just comfort me—it anchored me. My relationship with Jesus became a sacred space where I could be vulnerable, seen, and poured back into. It was only through this spiritual grounding that I found clarity, strength, and the confidence to rise, not just to survive menopause, but to thrive through it. I learned that healing starts not with doing more, but with releasing more—letting go of shame, perfectionism, and pressure, and leaning into divine grace. When you anchor your journey in faith, you don't just find healing... you find home. It was from my place of healing that everything else emerged: the message, the mission, and creating the Menopause Energized program.

Let This Prayer Wash Over You

Lord, I come to you carrying wounds I have held onto for far too long. I ask for the strength to forgive those who have hurt me, not because they deserve it, but because I deserve peace. Help me release the weight of anger, bitterness, and resentment that has kept me bound. Father, teach me how to forgive myself for the mistakes I've made and the moments I wish I could change. Remind me that your grace is bigger than my past, and your love reaches deeper than my regrets. Fill the empty spaces in my heart with your peace and guide me forward in freedom. Amen.

Affirmations for Spiritual Release and Renewal

1. I release what no longer serves my peace, and I open my heart to God's healing grace.

2. I am worthy of forgiveness, both from others and from myself.

3. Each day, I choose peace over bitterness and faith over fear.

4. God's grace covers my past, strengthens my present, and prepares my future.

5. I am no longer held captive by old wounds; I walk in freedom and favor.

Recognizing the Everyday Miracles and Blessings Around You

It's easy to get so caught up in the demands, struggles, and noise of daily life that we overlook the quiet, gentle ways when God shows up for us every single day. We often look for big, dramatic miracles — the healing, the financial breakthrough, the life-changing opportunity — and miss the countless small blessings happening all around us. A kind word from a stranger, the beauty of a sunrise, a moment of unexpected peace in the middle of a stressful day, or the steady beat of your own heart when life feels overwhelming... these are miracles too. God's presence isn't reserved for the extraordinary; it's woven into the ordinary moments we so often take for granted.

Recognizing these everyday miracles is not about pretending life is always perfect but about shifting our focus from what's missing to what's present. When you train your heart to notice the simple blessings — like laughter with a friend, the warmth of sunlight on your face, or a verse of scripture that speaks directly to what you're going through, you begin to realize just how active God's hand is in your life. Gratitude is a powerful spiritual tool. It keeps your heart open, softens your spirit, and reminds you that even in the small seasons, you are never forgotten. The more you look for his presence, the more you'll find it often in places you never expected.

Surrendering Control

One of the hardest lessons I've had to learn in my spiritual journey is that I am not in control—because God is, and his plans stretch far beyond what I can comprehend. As women, especially in midlife, we carry so much. We try to hold everything together for our families, our careers, our health, and our future. But no matter how hard we plan, life has a way of reminding us that some things are simply beyond our reach. It is a difficult truth to accept, especially when we have spent years believing that if we work hard enough, pray long enough, or worry just a little more, we can somehow prevent the hard things from happening. The real peace comes not in managing every outcome but in surrendering those outcomes to God and trusting that his plan, even when it doesn't match ours, is still good.

Surrendering does not mean giving up; it means letting go of the illusion of control and placing your trust in the one who sees the full picture when you only see a piece of it. It's choosing to believe that God is working behind the scenes in ways you can't yet see, and what feels like a setback might be setting you up for a comeback. I have learned to pray not just for the outcome I want, but for the wisdom to trust him, even if the answer is no or not yet. When we surrender control, we free ourselves from anxiety, fear, and constant tension. We open our hearts to peace, to growth, and to the beautiful, unexpected ways God shows up when we finally step aside and let him lead.

As we come to the close of this chapter, remember that your spiritual journey is uniquely filled with ups and downs, questions and revelations. It is okay to have moments of doubt, to wrestle with your faith, and to seek comfort in God in your own way and time. Through the storms and the stillness, the letting go and the holding on, God's presence remains a constant source of strength and hope. Embracing forgiveness, recognizing everyday blessings, surrendering control, and nurturing a daily connection with him are all steps toward a deeper, more resilient faith. May this journey inspire you to keep moving forward with grace. Walk in faith, trusting that even when the path feels uncertain, you are never alone.

Conclusion

Faith is not about having all the answers, but it's about trusting the unseen hand guiding your steps through every storm and season. In forgiveness, in surrender, in noticing the small miracles, and in the quiet moments of prayer, you are being shaped and strengthened in ways you cannot yet see. Remember, no matter how winding the path or how heavy the heart, God's presence is the steady light that never fades. Walk forward with courage, knowing you are deeply loved and never alone. As we move through the menopause journey, many of us will face challenges we didn't expect—physical symptoms, emotional waves, or even personal life storms that hit us when we're already feeling vulnerable. These moments can shake us, but they don't have to break us. It's okay to feel overwhelmed, but don't let those challenges knock you down so far that you forget your strength. Keep the faith. Lean on your inner resilience, your spiritual foundation, and the support around you. In the middle of the storm, you are being shaped, not defeated. Let faith carry you forward, one step at a time, beyond the Footprints of Menopause.

Affirmation: *"I give myself permission to pause, to breathe, and to heal. In stillness, I reconnect with my spirit, and in that connection, I find peace, strength, and restoration."*

CHAPTER 5
CARRYING THE HEALING FORWARD

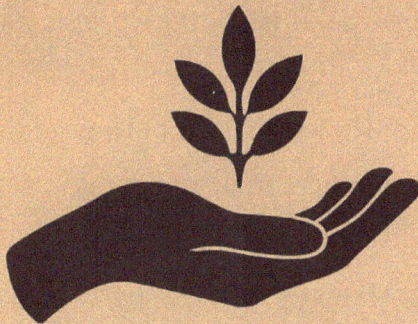

5 Carrying the Healing Forward: One Truthful Step at a Time

Healing is a journey made up of distinct but interconnected stages—each one essential to restoring balance and wholeness in our lives. Although presented in stages, healing is never strictly linear; it's a continuous, evolving process that requires patience, grace, and a willingness to revisit any stage as life unfolds. Together, these stages create a foundation for lasting transformation and renewed vitality.

This chapter is about giving yourself grace during your time of healing. It is about releasing guilt for stepping back, quieting the inner critic, and accepting that the path to wholeness is not always quick or neat. Healing is layered, personal, and deeply sacred, and this chapter will remind you that both the pauses and the progress are equally valuable parts of your journey.

Healing as a Way of Life: Walking Boldly into Your Next Chapter

It is time to carry that wisdom forward. With healing as your foundation, you are ready to step boldly into confidence and reveal the most radiant version of yourself. Healing was the doorway. Now, you walk the path. With clarity restored, inner strength renewed, and emotional burdens lifted, you are ready for the next chapter. Healing is not a one-time event or a destination you finally arrive at — it's an ongoing, evolving process. Life will always bring new challenges, transitions, and unexpected experiences that test your resilience and stir up old wounds. If you treat healing as something you only address when you're in crisis, you risk carrying unhealed hurts and suppressed emotions that quietly affect your peace, relationships, and decisions. Continuous healing enables you to remain emotionally and spiritually aligned, creating space for growth, forgiveness, and self-discovery as life unfolds. It's a way of tending to yourself with honesty and care, acknowledging that no matter how strong you are, you are still human and deserving of compassion in every season.

The importance of continuous healing lies in the fact that new experiences often reveal deeper layers of past pain or unresolved emotions we thought we'd moved past. Each new chapter of life — whether it's a relationship shift, career change, or personal loss — can uncover feelings that need attention. By making healing a regular part of your life, you remain emotionally clear, spiritually grounded, and open to life's lessons without becoming hardened by them. It is not about chasing perfection or never feeling pain again; it is about staying connected to yourself enough to recognize when it is time to pause, reflect, and heal a little more. That's where true wholeness lives — in the ongoing, gentle work of honoring your wounds while still choosing to rise.

It is one thing to acknowledge that healing is necessary, but it's another to be patient and kind to yourself while you are in the thick of it. Too often, we pressure ourselves to bounce back quickly or keep moving as if nothing happened. But true healing requires intention, rest, and permission to not be okay for a while. This is how you are able to walk boldly into the next chapter of your life.

Making Space for Your Own Healing

There's something deeply woven into the fabric of who we are as women—this instinct to nurture, to give, to care for everyone else before ourselves. But while showing up for others, we often forget the one person who needs us the most: we need ourselves. We carry so much. We move through challenges that demand strength, grace, and perseverance. Even when life feels heavy, we keep giving, keep showing up, keep holding space for others. But here's what we rarely say out loud—we need time to heal, too. It might not be the pain of losing a loved one or the pain of a broken relationship, but in caring for everyone else, we sometimes lose ourselves. That, too, is a kind of grief. That, too, deserves space.

So, this is your reminder, ladies: taking time to heal is not selfish, it's sacred. It is how we reconnect with who we are beneath the roles, the routines, and the responsibilities.

During my menopause journey, I never paused to ask myself if I was moving too fast. I just kept going on autopilot, making sure everyone else was okay, even though I was breaking down emotionally and physically. I was pouring from an empty cup. Then one day, I had a moment of clarity. I looked at myself and said, "Sheila, you need to take time out to heal. You've probably noticed I've repeated that phrase throughout this chapter. There's a reason for that. It is not just words; it is a truth we have to keep reminding ourselves until it finally sinks in. For those of us facing menopause with real intensity, like I did, healing is not an option; it is essential. The only way to make it through is to slow down, listen to what our bodies are saying, and give ourselves the time and space to heal.

It was not until I truly acknowledged the need to care for myself emotionally that everything began to shift. That is when I started asking, What brings me joy? What fuels my passion? What lights me up inside? And most importantly, what can I put into motion that feeds my soul? Sometimes, we don't recognize what's happening in our lives until we have hit rock bottom. And oddly enough, it is in that brokenness that something sacred happens—we wake up. We realize it is time to make a change. Walking through this menopause journey has taught me more about life than I could have ever imagined. And as I've mentioned before, I came out stronger, more grounded, and more confident on the other side. I was no longer just pushing my way through this season.

The Sacred Turning Point

Sometimes, the challenges we face in life are not meant to break us, but to awaken us. The challenges reveal a strength we never knew we possessed and open doors to paths we never imagined walking. What feels like a setback or a storm often becomes a sacred turning point, a moment that shifts your perspective, reshapes your priorities, and leads you toward a new, unexpected journey with deeper purpose and resilience. Had I not walked through this experience, I would have never gained the clarity to birth this book or the fire to create my Menopause Energized program. It was through my own struggles that purpose found me. Now, as a Menopause health coach, I have the privilege of guiding other women, not just to survive menopause, but to help them to rise, reclaim their power, and transform every part of their lives in the process.

It is a process of shedding old versions of yourself, releasing what no longer serves you, and slowly stepping into a new, healthier way of being. Along the way, there are different stages we are called to face: moments of reflection, release, restoration, and growth, each one preparing us for the next. True healing requires us to move through these layers with honesty and grace, because only by honoring each part of the process can we fully transform. It is not about racing to the finish line but about embracing the continuous unfolding of your journey, trusting that with every step, you are becoming stronger, wiser, and more whole.

Embracing the Pause: How Faith Became My First Step Toward Healing

So, someone might ask me, "Where did you begin when you finally decided to take time out to heal? What did it take to get there? My answer would be this: it started with embracing my spiritual journey. For those of us who believe, that means more than just quiet reflection; it's about leaning into the power of prayer, seeking peace in God's presence, and nurturing a personal relationship with Jesus. It's about creating space to listen, to surrender, and to be guided through the healing process, not by our strength, but by divine strength. That spiritual foundation became the first and most essential step, as I discussed in the previous chapter.

Emotional Healing

Once you've taken the time to reconnect with yourself spiritually — grounding your faith, restoring your inner peace, and finding meaning beyond the pain — the next step is to address the emotional wounds that linger. Spiritual healing lays the foundation, but emotional healing is where you unpack what you've been carrying: the grief, anger, fear, disappointment, and unspoken heartache. It's about learning to name your emotions, feel them without shame, and release what no longer serves you. Journaling, therapy, heartfelt conversations, and self-compassion practices are powerful tools during this stage. Emotional healing allows you to shed the heaviness of what was, so you can fully embrace the wholeness of who you are becoming.

Physical Healing

Once your spirit feels grounded and your emotions have been acknowledged and gently processed, your body often carries the residue of stress, trauma, or neglect that needs attention. Physical healing is about listening deeply to your body's needs—whether that means nourishing it with wholesome foods, moving in ways that feel good, prioritizing restful sleep, or seeking medical care when necessary. It's the practice of honoring your body as the vessel that supports your entire healing journey. Self-care routines become essential tools to restore energy, build strength, and maintain balance.

This stage also involves creating habits that support long-term wellness and vitality, because healing isn't complete without caring for the physical dimension of your being. When your body feels healthy and strong, it amplifies the healing you've done emotionally and spiritually, giving you more energy and resilience to fully embrace life's possibilities. This is carrying the healing forward.

Mental & Cognitive Healing

Once your spirit, emotions, and body have been tended to, it's essential to cultivate a healthy mental space. Healing the mind means becoming aware of negative thought patterns, limiting beliefs, or mental clutter that may hold you back from fully thriving. It involves intentionally replacing harmful or self-sabotaging thoughts with empowering, positive affirmations and developing mental habits that foster clarity, focus, and resilience. This can include mindfulness practices, meditation, learning new skills, reading uplifting content, or collaborating with a coach or therapist to reframe perspectives.

Mental healing helps you break free from cycles of doubt, fear, and confusion, allowing you to move forward with confidence and purpose. It also supports sustained emotional and physical well-being by reducing stress and improving your ability to cope with life's challenges.

Social & Community Healing

Healing isn't just an internal process — it's deeply influenced by the people and environment around us. Before the healing process begins, many of us find ourselves withdrawing from others and retreating into isolation. When pain, confusion, or overwhelming emotions take hold, it's natural to pull back to protect ourselves from further hurt or judgment. This solitude can feel like a safe space to gather our scattered pieces, but it can also deepen feelings of loneliness and disconnection. Isolation often acts as a barrier between us and the support we need, making it harder to move forward. Recognizing this tendency is an important first step because healing ultimately invites us to gently reengage with ourselves, with others, and with the world around us.

Social healing involves surrounding yourself with supportive, positive relationships that encourage your growth and well-being. It's about setting healthy boundaries, seeking connection with those who uplift you, and sometimes letting go of toxic relationships that drain your energy. Rebuilding trust, communication, and community can provide a powerful source of belonging and strength as you continue your healing journey.

Purpose and Identity Restoration

One of the most beautiful stages of healing is Purpose and Identity Restoration — the moment you begin to rediscover who you are beyond the pain you've carried. So often, trauma, loss, or difficult seasons cause us to lose touch with ourselves. Our identities become tied to what we've been through instead of who we truly are at our core. This stage invites you to peel back the layers of hurt, roles, and expectations to reconnect with the authentic version of yourself. It's about asking, *Who am I now? What truly matters to me?* Allow the answers to emerge without judgment. In this space, you begin to realize that while your past shaped you, it doesn't define you. The pain might have written a few chapters, but it doesn't get to author the rest of your story.

As you reclaim your identity, a renewed sense of purpose often rises to the surface. This may look like embracing new passions, setting fresh goals, or pursuing dreams you once set aside. You may feel called to help others, create something meaningful, or simply live with more intention and joy. The restoration of purpose gives new meaning to your experiences and reminds you that even broken places can become sacred ground for growth. It's a powerful affirmation that life after struggle isn't just about surviving — it's about thriving, evolving, and becoming the woman you were always meant to be.

Healing and Relationships

Healing doesn't just transform you; it transforms your relationships with the people you love. As you begin to release old pain, set healthier boundaries, and speak your truth, the dynamic with those closest to you naturally shifts. You become clearer about what you need, more present in your connections, and less willing to carry what was never yours to hold. Some relationships deepen because of your healing, while others may fall away as you outgrow old patterns. Either way, healing invites you to build relationships rooted in honesty, respect, and mutual care, not obligation or unspoken resentment. It teaches you to love from a place of wholeness, not from your wounds.

Ongoing Maintenance and Growth

Healing isn't something you arrive at and declare finished; it's a lifelong commitment to caring for yourself with honesty, compassion, and intention. You should periodically check in with yourself, acknowledge how life's changes affect you, and give yourself the space to process new emotions as they arise. It's about practicing self-reflection, asking what you need in each season, and allowing yourself to evolve. This stage reminds us that even when we feel whole, life will continue to present challenges, and the strength we build in our healing journey equips us to navigate those moments with grace and resilience.

Growth doesn't happen all at once; it's a gradual unfolding that requires patience and consistent care. Committing to ongoing maintenance might involve setting healthy boundaries, nurturing your physical and emotional wellness, feeding your mind with uplifting content, or surrounding yourself with people who support your growth. It also means extending grace to yourself when old wounds resurface or when setbacks occur, because healing isn't a straight line. This stage is not about chasing perfection but about embracing progress and understanding that every step you take to nurture your heart, mind, body, and spirit shapes the empowered, evolving woman you are becoming.

Loving Yourself through the Process

One of the most overlooked parts of healing is learning how to love yourself while you're still in the thick of it. It's easy to offer yourself kindness when everything feels good, but the real work happens when you choose to embrace the messy, unfinished, and uncertain parts of who you are. I had to learn how to look at the woman in the mirror — tired, frustrated, sometimes unsure — and still see someone worth loving. Not because I was perfect or had it all figured out, but because I was doing my best, continuing to move forward, and refusing to abandon myself. In those moments, I realized that self-love isn't a reward you earn at the end of the journey; it's something you give yourself in the middle of it. It is found in the quiet decisions to rest, to say no, to forgive yourself, and to celebrate small victories no one else sees. The more I extended grace to myself, the lighter the load became, and the clearer my sense of worth grew. Healing taught me that loving yourself isn't selfish — it's survival, and it's the foundation for every good thing that follows. Healing taught me that my strength was never in how much I could carry, but in how willing I was to finally lay things down. It showed me that it's okay to step back, to feel, to unravel, and to rebuild on my own terms. What I thought would break me reshaped me. And in the quiet moments away from titles, expectations, and the constant need to be everything for everyone, I met a version of myself I didn't even know I was missing.

Healing was not about reclaiming my past self—it was about becoming someone new. I healed to become someone wiser, softer in spirit, stronger in boundaries, and clearer in purpose. The lessons weren't always easy, but they were necessary. Now, I move through life with intention, honoring both where I've been and where I'm headed. I've learned that healing isn't about returning to the old version of myself; it's about creating a new, unapologetic, beautiful whole one.

Conclusion

Healing is one of the most personal, sacred journeys a woman can take. It requires courage to face yourself honestly, to acknowledge what's been buried, and faith to believe that you're worthy of peace, wholeness, and joy on the other side of it. This journey isn't about erasing your past or pretending the pain didn't happen; it is about gathering wisdom from every experience and using it to shape the strongest, truest version of your future self. As you move through each stage, you'll uncover new layers of resilience, clarity, and strength that you may not have known existed within you.

In the end, healing isn't just about feeling better; it is about becoming better for yourself. It's a commitment to rise each day with intention, choosing growth over stagnation and hope over defeat. This process is your own to shape and to honor in your own time and way. And while no one else can walk it for you, you're never walking it alone. Every footprint forward is a quiet declaration that you are reclaiming your life, your voice, and your power, and that is a beautiful, unstoppable thing.

Affirmation: *"I give myself permission to heal fully, gently, and at my own pace, knowing I am worthy of peace, wholeness, and joy as I move forward into my next chapter.*

CHAPTER 6
SOUL NOURISHMENT

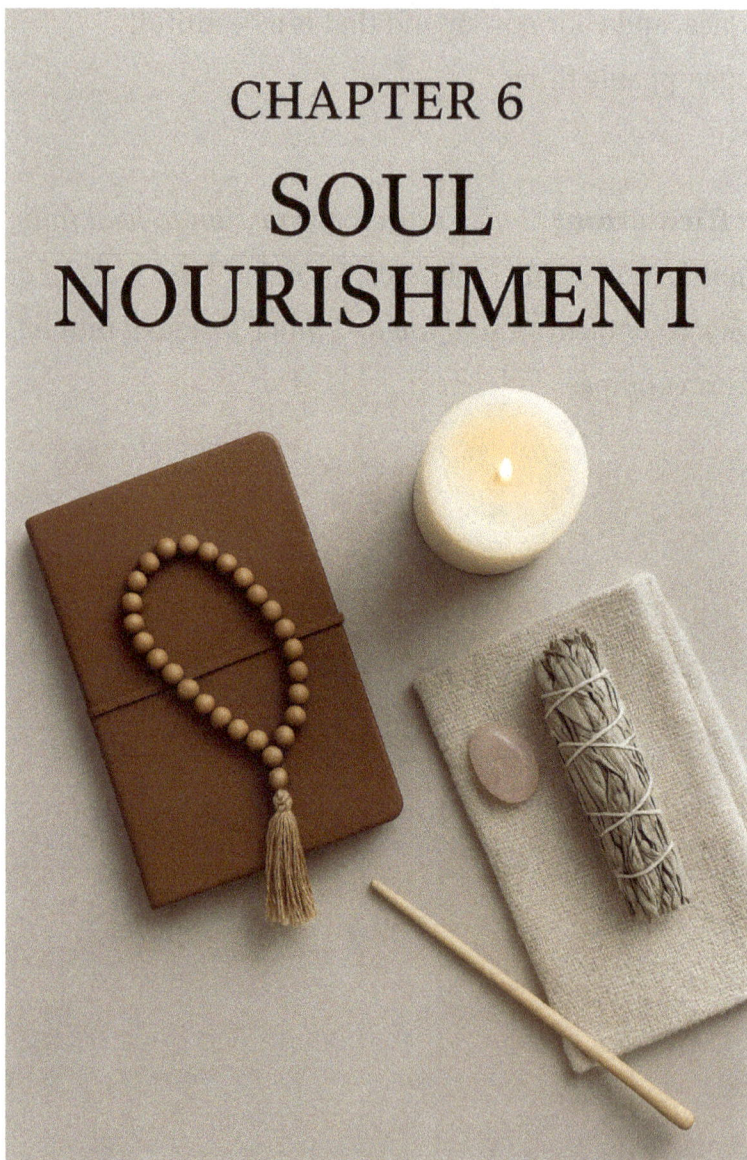

6 Soul Nourishment: Listening to the Parts We've Silenced

While a spiritual journey is about deepening your relationship with God — walking in faith, growing spiritually, and aligning with divine purpose — soul searching is a more personal and reflective process. It's the quiet inner work of asking who you truly are, what you deeply desire, and what's missing or misaligned in your life.

During menopause, many women experience an unexpected sense of disconnection — not just from their faith, but from their bodies, joy, and creativity. The shifting of hormones that cause emotional highs and lows, and physical changes, can create a fog that dulls the things that once lit them up inside. Prayers may feel distant, laughter becomes rare, and creative outlets they once loved gather dust. It's easy to lose touch with spiritual practices, the hobbies that once made hours fly by, or the simple pleasures that used to spark genuine joy. This disconnection isn't a flaw — it's a natural response to the overwhelming internal transformation menopause brings. But it's also a gentle signal from the soul that it's time to reach for those anchors again.

The Personal Meaning of Soul

What do you think about when you hear the word soul? No dictionary definitions—what does the word truly mean to you? To me, it means a feeling of being connected to something—positive or negative—that I cannot see. It's a sensation of happiness or sadness, a sense of belonging, a deep burning feeling, whether uplifting or painful. It's a sense of being either lost or fully known—a mysterious force that shapes who I am.

As I journey through menopause, I've never felt more deeply connected to my soul than I do now. My soul connects me and takes me to places I've never been before. It speaks to my inner life—my faith, intuition, and emotional depth—and guides me beyond physical. It's less about geography and more about internal landscapes: new levels of understanding, healing, creativity, and spiritual intimacy.

Have you ever heard the saying, My soul cries out? Sometimes I wonder—do we really know what our soul cries out for? Is it a connection to God, or divine wisdom that opens your heart in ways you've never experienced?

The Healing Dimensions of our Soul

The first is the Grounded Soul — Our Connection to Earth and Body

This is the part that craves safety, ritual, and rest. It anchors us in the present moment and whispers, *"You belong here."* It's where our nervous system finds peace and where somatic practices become sacred.

The Wild Soul — Our Passion, Instinct, and Desire

This is the untamed spirit within. It holds our anger, our sensuality, and our intuition. It's where truth roars and creativity flows. Ignoring this aspect often leads to burnout because this is where our vitality lives.

The Reflective Soul — Our Emotional Depth and Inner Knowing is the soul's journal keeper. It watches, listens, feels, and remembers. It's where self-compassion blooms and where we process both pain and joy.

The Visionary Soul — Our Purpose, Dreams, and Higher Wisdom. This part carries our calling. It's the one who dreams beyond circumstances and sees potential in everything. It seeks alignment with something greater—our higher self, spirit, legacy, or divine mystery.

The Healing Soul — Our Resilience, Forgiveness, and Self-Compassion. This is the part that stitches us back together. It grieves, releases, reconciles, and rebuilds. It knows that wholeness isn't perfection—it's integration.

When the Soul Goes Quiet: A Hole in my Soul

When the soul is struggling, it's as if each layer is dimmed by silence and overwhelm. *The Grounded Soul* feels displaced, restless in a body it no longer recognizes, disconnected from the rhythms that once brought peace. *The Wild Soul* grows quiet, its passions buried under fatigue and the weight of caretaking, whispering needs that go unmet. *The Reflective Soul* wrestles with self-doubt, replaying old narratives of failure or invisibility. *The Visionary Soul* loses clarity, unsure of its purpose or path, as dreams fade beneath daily demands. *The Healing Soul*—the part meant to mend—can feel frozen, unable to begin the work because it has not been given permission to feel. In this state, she's surviving on autopilot, but inside there's a quiet ache: a longing to remember who she truly is.

There were seasons in my life when I felt like I was moving through the world with a hole in my soul—an emptiness I couldn't name but felt in every quiet moment. I would show up smiling, carry the weight, and follow through on what had to be done... but underneath it all, something was missing. It was as if pieces of me had slowly slipped away in the giving, the enduring, and the adjusting. I didn't feel broken, exactly—I felt hollow. Only when I paused long enough to listen to that silence and to acknowledge what I had neglected in myself, did the true healing begin. That hole wasn't a flaw; it was a call, A longing to be nourished, seen, and reclaimed.

Signs the Soul Is Starving

When the soul is starving, it doesn't always scream — sometimes, it quietly aches in the background of your life. You might feel an unexplainable emptiness, even when everything on the outside appears fine. There's a lingering restlessness, a sense that something is missing, though you can't quite name it. Joy feels fleeting, connections feel shallow, and you find yourself going through the motions rather than truly living. It shows up in the chronic fatigue that no amount of sleep can fix, the irritability you can't explain, or the constant search for distraction to avoid sitting still with yourself. These are signs your soul is hungry for deeper meaning, authentic connection, and a return to what truly nourishes you from within.

When your soul is starving, the small, beautiful moments of life pass by unnoticed — a sunset becomes just a sky, a smile from a stranger feels insignificant, and the things that once sparked joy now feel like obligations. You lose your sense of purpose and passion, often feeling disconnected from your own voice and intuition. This depletion can manifest as anxiety, burnout, and a deep longing for something more, even if you can't articulate what that 'more' is. Recognizing these signs is not a weakness —

it's an invitation to pause, listen, and begin the gentle, vital work of feeding your soul again.

The Meaning of Soul Nourishment

Soul nourishment is the intentional act of feeding the deepest parts of ourselves, not with food, but with meaning, connection, and restoration. It is about tending to the emotional, spiritual, and energetic layers of who we are, especially during seasons of transition like menopause. Just as the body requires rest and nourishment, the soul craves nourishment in the form of reflection, compassion, and beauty. It craves rituals that honor our truth, spaces that allow us to exhale, and messages that remind us that we are more than our roles, symptoms, or responsibilities.

In the menopause journey, soul nourishment becomes essential, not optional. It is how we reclaim the parts of ourselves that may have been buried under years of giving, striving, and coping. Through reflective practices, storytelling, creative expression, and connection with others, we begin to feel full again, not just in our bodies, but in our purpose. We remember that thriving is not about doing more, it is about being more present, more honest, and more tender with ourselves. Soul nourishment is how we come home to who we have always been, and who we are still becoming.

Rest as a Ritual

Soul nourishment is a form of rest that goes beyond closing your eyes—it's the kind of renewal that sinks into your spirit. It's the moment you pause not just to recharge your energy, but to reconnect with your essence. Sleep may quiet the body, but soul-nourishing rest quiets the noise inside you—the relentless expectations, emotional fatigue, and spiritual disconnection. It's found in spaces where you feel safe enough to exhale fully, to let go, and to be tender with yourself. Whether it's through reflection, ritual, creativity, or stillness, this kind of rest repairs the unseen tears in your spirit and reminds you that healing isn't a task—it's a state of being.

Uplifted by Connection

Soul nourishment is not found in mere presence—it's found in meaningful connection. It's not about being surrounded by people, but about being seen, heard, and felt in your truth. A company can fill a room, but connection fills a heart. When we're deeply witnessed by someone who holds space for our story without fixing or judging, we rise a little. We soften, exhale, and begin to heal. This kind of connection uplifts because it affirms that our experience matters. In the menopause journey, especially where so much can feel isolated, true connection becomes a sanctuary. It restores dignity, deepens self-trust, and reminds us that we're walking a shared path—and we don't have to walk it alone.

Awakened by Truth, Touched by Beauty

When weariness settles deep—not just in the muscles but in the spirit—it isn't caffeine or distraction that revives us. It's the truth that clears the fog and gives shape to what we've been carrying. It's beauty that reminds us of joy, wonder, and our capacity to feel, and it's meaning that reawakens the why behind it all. Soul nourishment is found when these three forces converge: when a sunset speaks directly to your ache, when an honest conversation lifts a hidden burden, and when you suddenly remember that your life is still full of purpose. In the menopause journey, these moments aren't luxuries—they are lifelines. They restore not just energy, but aliveness.

Nourishing your soul during menopause means intentionally creating space to reconnect with what makes you feel alive and spiritually whole. It could be as simple as sitting quietly with a sunrise, journaling prayers or thoughts without judgment, or picking up a creative project you left behind. Surrounding yourself with women who remind you of your worth, seeking out lighthearted moments, and embracing small rituals of gratitude can help rekindle that spark. This season isn't about returning to who you were before, but about rediscovering new, soulful ways to experience faith, joy, and creativity as the woman you are now — wiser, deeper, and still beautifully capable of wonder.

The Soul-Nourishing Toolkit

The Soul-Nourishing Toolkit is a collection of simple, yet powerful practices designed to help you reconnect with your inner self and cultivate a deep sense of peace and fulfillment. It's about creating daily rituals that feed your spirit, whether through mindful breathing, journaling your thoughts and feelings, or spending time in nature to awaken your senses. This toolkit encourages you to slow down, listen to your intuition, and honor your emotional needs without judgment. By regularly tuning into these practices, you build resilience against stress and find a steady source of comfort through life's transitions.

1. *Speak Life Over Yourself-* We have all done it — whispered harsh words to ourselves in moments of insecurity: "I'm not enough." "I'm too old." "I should be further along." But these are not the words of truth. They're echoes of wounds, not reflections of who you really are. Your words matter. Replace negative self-talk with truth: "I am loved." I am healing." God is guiding me." Your words matter — more than you think. Every thought you speak over yourself becomes a seed planted in the soil of your soul. You may not notice it, but every choice plants either fear or faith, shame or grace, defeat or strength.

2. *Ask Yourself Deeper Questions-* What am I pretending to be okay with? What did I need but didn't get? What would my life look like if I honored my true self? It asks you to get honest about the places where you've been tolerating, enduring, or smiling through situations that are actually hurting or draining you. Are you pretending exhaustion is normal? Are you pretending the relationship doesn't hurt? Are you pretending the role you're playing still fits, when deep down, it doesn't? Sometimes we convince ourselves that it's fine because speaking the truth feels too risky. Soul nourishment begins the moment we stop pretending and start acknowledging what's really going on inside.

3. *Reconnect with Your Inner Voice-*Your inner voice is often drowned out by noise — social media, to-do lists, and other people's opinions. Create moments of stillness in your day. Morning silence with coffee before the world wakes up. A quiet walk without your phone. Sitting in your car before going inside. Write freely. Let the pen move without editing your thoughts. Pay attention to the things that make you

feel aligned, lifted, or deeply peaceful. These moments often echo your inner voice saying, "This is right for you." If you have ignored or silenced your inner voice for years, don't shame yourself. This is a reunion, not a punishment. Be kind and curious with yourself, not critical.

4. *Honor Your Truth Without Apology-* Say no without guilt. Rest without earning it. You don't need to shrink, soften, or explain your truth to make others comfortable. You don't need to apologize for needing space, for changing your mind, or for no longer carrying what you were never meant to hold. We have been taught that saying no is selfish. That resting is lazy. That our worth is tied to how much we do and how little we ask for. But healing begins when you stop performing for approval and start honoring your truth. Rest without earning it. You don't have to be exhausted to deserve a break. You don't need to prove your worth through hustle or sacrifice. Your value isn't tied to productivity — it's tied to your existence. Feel what you feel, without shame. You don't have to smile through or at everything. You don't have to be the strong one all

the time. You can grieve. You can be angry. You can be unsure. Honoring your truth means allowing all of you to exist, not just the parts that look polished

5. *Find Beauty That Speaks to You-* Visit a museum, listen to music, and read poetry. Maybe even write your own poetry that reflects on the past and the future of your journey. It is not about being creative; it's about expressing the emotions your heart has been holding quietly for far too long.

6. *Release Roles You've Outgrown-* Are you clinging to identities that no longer serve you? "The fixer, "the strong one, "the silent one." Sometimes we stay in these roles because they once protected us, but now they're suffocating who we're becoming. Letting go is not failure — it's freedom.

7. *Let Yourself Grieve What Was-* Not everything we lost is bad. Not everything we miss is meant to return. Grief isn't just for death — it's for the versions of you that no longer fit, the seasons that ended before you were ready, and the dreams that didn't unfold the way you hoped. Let yourself mourn them. Some things had to fall away for you to grow. That old relationship.

That former role. That identity you clung to. It served you once, but now it's asking to be released. Not everything we miss is meant to return. Missing something doesn't mean you need it back. It just reflects that it had significance. Honoring that truth is part of soul nourishment.

8. *Stop Performing, Start Feeling-* Are you trying to look healed more than being healed? Try not to put on a show for others — your healing is not a performance. But I know you don't want to look broken down either, like you're fishing for sympathy. The goal is not to hide or to overshare — it's to honor what you're feeling without pretending and without performing. You can be honest without being exposed, and vulnerable without being pitied.

9. *Choose What Fuels Your Energy-* Not Just Your Schedule. Ask: Does this replenish me or just keep me busy? We live in a world that rewards productivity but rarely asks whether we're being *nourished* in the process. Many of us have calendars full of responsibilities; appointments, meetings, errands, and obligations — but we still feel emotionally and

spiritually empty at the end of the day. Busyness can be a mask for avoidance or a way we prove our worth to others. But the truth is: not everything that fills your schedule feeds your soul. Start paying attention to the things that give you energy versus those that drain you. This is about being intentionally selfish. You are not here to prove yourself by running on empty. You are here to live fully, joyfully, and on purpose.

There were days when I would say yes when I wanted to say no. There were times when my calendar was full, believing that being busy meant being valuable— but all it really did was drain me. It took time, honesty, and some painful unlearning to realize that I was keeping myself occupied but not truly fulfilled. This journey has taught me that healing is not just about slowing down — it's about choosing what nourishes my soul. I had to learn to stop performing and start listening... to God, my body, and my inner self. In the process, I uncovered a peace from within that had been quietly missing from my life.

Conclusion

Soul nourishment starts when you permit yourself to be honest, even if it's messy. Soul nourishment often means shedding, not adding, creating without performing, and reconnecting you to your true self. Soul nourishment is about feeding the deepest part of yourself — the part that craves meaning, peace, and connection beyond the physical. When we make space to care for our inner world, we strengthen our resilience, renew our energy, and reconnect with what truly matters.

At its core, the Soul-Nourishing Toolkit isn't a one-size-fits-all solution — it's a personalized set of tools that resonate with you and your unique journey. These practices help transform moments of overwhelm into opportunities for growth and self-discovery. Embracing your toolkit invites you to nurture your whole being — mind, body, and soul — especially during a transition like menopause when your inner balance is more important than ever.

Affirmation: *"My soul craves connection, peace, meaning, and renewal—and I honor that hunger with gentleness. I choose what nourishes my spirit, strengthens my heart, and draws me closer to the life "I was made to live—not just exist."*

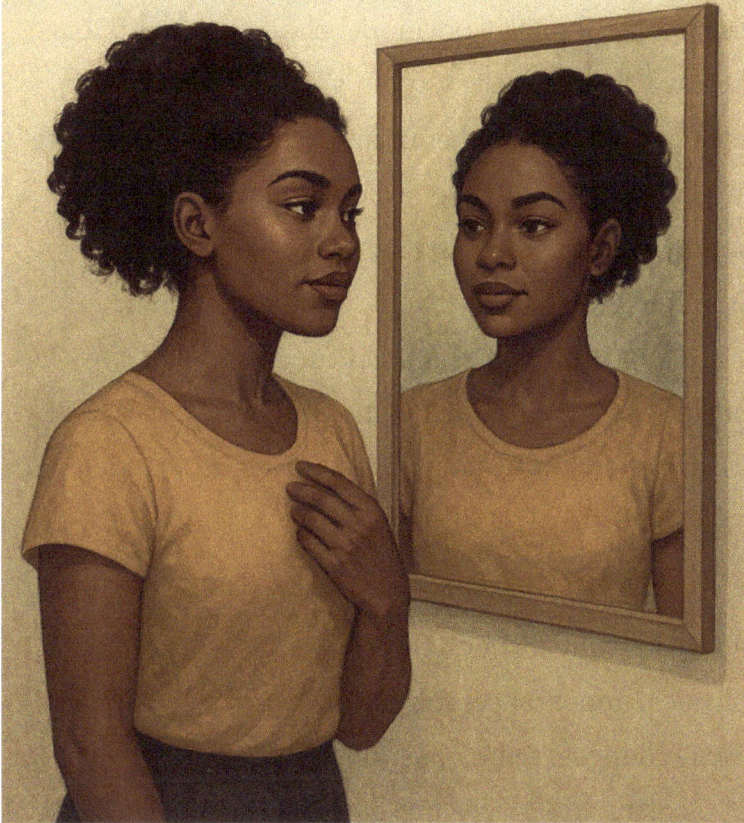

CHAPTER 7
Confidence In The Mirror

7 Confidence in the Mirror

Along this journey, many of us will begin to question our worth, wondering if we're still enough, still valuable, still significant in this season of life. We'll ask ourselves: Am I still beautiful? Do I still matter? Is my presence still powerful? These quiet, aching questions deserve honest, soul-affirming answers.

During menopause, hormonal changes can influence how we view ourselves, often affecting mood, memory, energy, and emotional resilience. When we are going through the emotional phase of the journey, some of us become more sensitive to criticism — whether it's from others or from that harsh inner voice — it is often because the identity is shifting, the hormones are amplifying emotional responses, and we are questioning parts of ourselves we once felt solid in. It's real, it's tender, and it deserves compassion.

As we journey through the menopausal years, our physical appearance may naturally shift—and with those changes, quiet questions can arise within us. Am I still attractive? Does my skin still carry the radiant glow it once did? These reflections are not signs of vanity, but invitations to rediscover our beauty in a deeper, more soulful way. The truth is, your worth is not measured by age, appearance, or the roles you've outgrown. It's rooted in who you are at your core — a woman of wisdom, resilience, and undeniable strength. This chapter is not about fading; it is about rising into a version of yourself that's freer, bolder, and unapologetically whole. You are and have always been enough.

The Many Faces of Self-Worth: Understanding What Really Defines You

You will often hear words like self-worth, self-esteem, self-image, self-confidence, and self-compassion used interchangeably, but while they may sound similar, each carries its own unique meaning. To truly reclaim the confidence, you see in the mirror, it is essential first to understand how these concepts differ and what each one reveals about your relationship with yourself. Only then can we begin the deeper work of healing and rebuilding the confidence that radiates from within.

Self-Worth

Self-worth is your overall belief in your value as a person — simply because you exist — not tied to job titles, accomplishments, or comparisons. If a woman believed she was unlovable, undeserving of respect, or worthless as a person, this would fall under low self-worth. Self-worth is the belief that you deserve love, respect, and good things in life. In the menopausal years, some women will go through a period of feeling like they are not valuable and do not deserve the good things in life. For decades, women have been taught — subtly and openly — that their worth is tied to their youth, appearance, productivity, caregiving roles, or their ability to meet others' needs. When those external markers shift (through aging, career changes, empty nests, or changing bodies), it can trigger a crisis of identity. An example is: "I'm not good enough as a person, no matter what I do."

On top of that, hormonal changes during menopause can impact mood, emotional resilience, and self-perception, making it easier for old insecurities and limiting beliefs to resurface. Emotional wounds, unresolved traumas, and years of putting yourself last can quietly erode a woman's sense of worth.

The path to healing begins when you choose to believe in your self-worth. When you start recognizing that your value is constant and reclaim the parts of yourself you may have lost along the way, you open the door to real emotional freedom. Honoring your true self — not the version the world told you to be, means acknowledging, accepting, and embracing who you truly are at your core, beyond titles, roles, expectations, and limitations placed on you by others or by yourself. It's about listening to your own voice, trusting your instincts, and making choices that align with your values, needs, and desires — not just what's expected of you. Honoring your true self means:

1.No longer shrinking to make others comfortable.
2. Speaking up for what you need and believe in.
3. Letting go of outdated labels and roles you've outgrown.
4. Allowing yourself to evolve without guilt or apology.
5. Making room for joy, peace, and experiences that nurture your spirit.

When you honor your true self, you stop seeking external validation and start trusting your own worth, wisdom, and intuition. This is when real freedom and confidence begin.

Self-Esteem

Self-esteem goes far beyond looking in the mirror at external features; it is just one layer of a much deeper landscape. It is how you judge your own capability, assertiveness, and the belief that you can handle what life throws your way. It's the quiet confidence that grows from experience, the inner voice that says, "I've got this," even when the path is uncertain. It's reflected in how you speak up for yourself, how you make decisions, and how you recover from setbacks—not because you're flawless, but because you trust your ability to learn, adapt, and move forward. Self-esteem is how you evaluate yourself based on your abilities, accomplishments, and how you believe others perceive you. It's the opinion you hold about yourself, influenced by your successes, failures, and experiences. Low self-esteem often focuses on your flaws and mistakes while overlooking your strengths and accomplishments.

Here is a good example: "I'm not going to get this promotion; Jean is a much better worker than I am. I'm just not smart enough." Self-esteem is about how you evaluate your abilities, qualities, and values in specific areas of your life.

Some women go through seasons of low self-esteem, especially during the menopausal years, because so much of their identity has been shaped by external expectations. Old insecurities and buried beliefs about feeling like you don't quite measure up can resurface as well. Society's obsession with youth and appearance only adds to this, making some women feel invisible or less valuable as they age. Low self-esteem in these seasons is often the result of years of unmet emotional needs, self-neglect, and giving away too much of yourself without replenishing your own spirit.

How Women Can Build Their Self-Esteem During Menopause

1. *Acknowledge and Accept the Changes*

Recognize that menopause brings natural physical, emotional, and hormonal shifts. Accepting these changes without judgment allows you to treat yourself with compassion instead of criticism.

2. *Challenge Negative Self-Talk*

Pay attention to the inner voice that may be critical or doubtful. When negative thoughts arise, question their truth and replace them with positive, affirming statements about your worth and abilities. When a negative thought like "I'm too old to start something new" arises, pause and challenge it. Ask yourself: Is this really true? What evidence do I have that age limits my ability to grow or succeed? "Then replace it with a powerful, affirming statement like I am full of wisdom and experience. My age gives me strength and perspective that younger people don't have. I have everything I need to learn, grow, and create new opportunities right now.

3. *Focus on Strengths and Achievements*

Reflect on your life experiences, skills, and qualities that make you unique. Instead of measuring yourself by flaws or fears, start tracking your wins — big or small. Every nourishing choice, every boundary honored, every moment of grace under pressure is a quiet triumph worth celebrating. Shift your gaze from what's missing to what's growing: your resilience, your wisdom, your ability to rise again. Self-esteem blooms when you recognize the strength in your story. Celebrate the wisdom and resilience you've gained over the years.

4. *Set Realistic Meaningful Goals*

Create small, achievable goals that align with your current values and passions. Accomplishing these goals builds confidence and a sense of purpose. When goals are too large, too fast, or disconnected from your present reality, they can set you up for disappointment. Repeated setbacks may chip away at your self-esteem, leaving you feeling incapable or defeated. Instead, honor your pace. Let each small win become a stepping stone toward something greater— because sustainable confidence is built one aligned step at a time.

5. Unfollow the Comparison Trap

Stop measuring yourself against others. Set goals that feel attainable and aligned with your own path. When you try to chase someone else's pace, you risk overwhelming yourself and slipping into self-doubt or low self-esteem. Stay focused on your growth — your only real competition is who you were yesterday. It means you're in motion — learning, shifting, shedding what no longer serves, and stepping more into who you are becoming. You were not meant to be a carbon copy of who you were yesterday.

6. Practice Self-Care and Prioritize Well-Being

Invest time in activities that nurture your body, mind, and spirit — like exercise, meditation, hobbies, or social connection. Feeling physically and emotionally cared for, supports a positive self-image.

6. Surround Yourself with Supportive People

Connect with friends, family, or support groups that uplift and encourage you. Sharing your experiences with others who understand and can validate your feelings and boost your confidence.

7. Learn and Grow

Engage in new learning or creative pursuits. Expanding your knowledge or skills can refresh your sense of self-esteem and reinforce your value beyond past roles.

8. Seek Professional Support if Needed

Therapists, coaches, or counselors can provide valuable tools and guidance to help individuals rebuild their self-esteem and navigate emotional challenges.

The good news is that self-esteem can be rebuilt. It begins by reconnecting with your worth, redefining your value beyond roles and appearance, and nurturing a kinder, more compassionate relationship with yourself.

Self-Confidence

Self-confidence is the belief in your ability to handle life's challenges and trust in your skills, choices, and judgments. It reflects how secure you feel when stepping into new situations, making decisions, or expressing yourself. Confidence grows through experience and can be rebuilt when shaken. Think of it as: I trust myself to navigate what's in front of me.

A woman with self-confidence might walk into a meeting knowing that while she may not have all the answers, she trusts in her ability to contribute something valuable. Even if she's nervous, she reminds herself, "I've prepared for this, and my perspective matters." When someone disagrees with her, she doesn't shrink back or take it personally; instead, she listens, responds calmly, and stands by her ideas. Self-confidence shows up in the way you carry yourself, make decisions, and take on new challenges — not because you think you are perfect, but because you believe in your ability to learn, grow, and handle whatever comes your way. In self-confidence, a person can feel very confident in specific skills or roles but can still have low self-esteem. For example, a woman might feel highly confident in her role as a professional—she knows she's skilled, articulate, and capable at work. She can lead meetings, solve problems, and mentor others with ease. But outside of that role, she may struggle with self-esteem. She might feel unworthy of love, question her appearance, or doubt her value when she's not "performing" or being productive. Her confidence is situational, tied to what she does—not who she is. See the difference?

How Women Can Build Their Self-Confidence During Menopause

1. Name the Loss, Then Reframe It

Confidence often dips when identity feels shaken — I don't recognize myself anymore. Start by acknowledging what's changed (physically, emotionally, relationally). Then ask: What new strengths are emerging? Maybe it's deeper empathy, sharper boundaries, or a clearer sense of what matters.

2. Rewire the Inner Dialogue

Menopause can amplify the inner critic: "I'm not sharp anymore," "I've lost my edge. "Practice gentle self-talk: "I'm learning to trust this new version of me. Use affirmations like: "I am evolving, not disappearing."

3. Reclaim Body Trust

Reconnect with your body — not as an object to fix, but as a partner to listen to. Gentle movement (like yoga, walking, or dancing) can rebuild the sense of I'm still strong. I'm still here. Nourishment, rest, and pleasure become acts of self-respect, not indulgence.

4. Set Micro-Goals and Celebrate Wins

Confidence grows through action, not by waiting to feel ready. Start small: record a voice note, post thoughts, try a new tech tool. Celebrate each step: I kept going even when I wanted to quit. That deserves to be noticed.

5. Surround Yourself with Reflective Mirrors

Spend time with people who see your power, not just your past. Join communities (like your coaching circles) where vulnerability is strength. Let others remind you of who you are when you forget.

6. Create a Symbolic Ritual

Confidence isn't just cognitive — it's emotional and symbolic. Consider a Reclamation Ritual: write a letter to your past self, burn limiting beliefs, or design a visual that represents your new chapter.

Self-Compassion

Self-compassion is the practice of extending the same kindness, care, and understanding to yourself that you would offer to a close friend in a moment of struggle. It means recognizing that being imperfect, failing, or experiencing difficulty is part of the shared human experience, not a reason to feel isolated or ashamed. Some women experiencing menopause, maintain compassion for others but may not direct the same compassion toward themselves.

Menopause can feel like a betrayal of the body and the familiar identity women have spent years building, when that sense of stability crumbles, self-compassion is often the first to fade. Many women are conditioned to be caregivers and to show up for others, no matter what. So, when menopause brings mood swings, brain fog, or physical changes, the instinct is often to push through rather than pause and offer yourself grace.

There's also a deeper emotional layer: when women feel they're "not performing" at their usual level—whether in work, relationships, or even self-care—they may judge themselves harshly. That inner critic gets louder, while the compassionate voice gets drowned out. Women are still expected to hold it all together; they may feel guilty for needing rest, support, or space to feel. But here's the truth: self-compassion isn't weakness—it is wisdom, and menopause is the perfect time to reclaim it.

Everyday Acts of Self-Compassion: Small Rituals That Rekindle Inner Kindness

1. Speak to Yourself Like a Friend

When self-criticism creeps in, pause and ask: Would I say this to someone I love? Replace harsh inner dialogue with gentle affirmations like: I'm doing the best I can with what I have today.

2. Practice Mirror Kindness

Look into the mirror and offer a soft smile or a kind word—even if it feels awkward at first. Try saying, You're still here, You're still worthy. It's not vanity—it's visibility.

3. Keep a Compassion Journal

Each evening, jot down one moment you showed up for yourself—or wish you had. Over time, this builds awareness and rewires the brain toward kindness. If you skip an evening, it's no big deal. Remember, we are not in this phase to beat ourselves up.

4. *Create a Self-Compassion Ritual*

Light a candle, sip tea, or take a mindful walk while repeating a mantra like I am allowed to rest. I am allowed to feel. Rituals anchor compassion in the body, not just the mind.

5. *Write a Forgiveness Letter to Yourself*

Acknowledge regrets or perceived failures with honesty and grace. End with: I forgive myself for not knowing what I didn't know then. I actually have not tried this one yet, but I speak it frequently.

6. *Surround Yourself with Reflective Souls*

Spend time with people who mirror your strength, not your self-doubt. Join a circle, support group, or coaching space where vulnerability is honored. I had and still have great mentors that has helped me through this phase of my life tremendously.

7. Celebrate Micro-Wins

You chose a nourishing breakfast instead of skipping the meal—celebrate that. You paused to take three deep breaths before reacting—honor that moment of self-awareness. You said "no" to something that drained you—recognize that boundary as a win. These micro-wins may seem small, but they are powerful signals that you're showing up for yourself, one choice at a time.

Self-compassion is the practice of treating yourself with the same kindness, understanding, and support that you would offer a dear friend — especially in moments of struggle, failure, or self-doubt. In essence, self-compassion invites you to meet your pain with presence and your imperfections with grace. It's not about self-pity or indulgence; it is about creating a nurturing inner environment where healing and growth can take root.

Conversations with Myself: The Power of Self-Reflection

What do all these tips have in common? They're rooted in self-reflection—the most powerful tool for navigating the menopausal season, however long it lasts. I've embraced so many of these practices that I find talking to myself constantly. My husband always asked if I was okay, and I smiled, and I would say to him, this is called self-reflecting, so I can support everything I love without crumbling. That depth is where transformation begins.

When All the Selves Speak: The Foundation of Wholeness

Menopause is not just a biological transition—it's a complete identity reorganization. That's why rebuilding and reinforcing the different "selves," like self-image, self-esteem, self-concept, and self-compassion, is so essential during this time. As hormones shift and bodies change, many women feel like strangers to themselves. The beliefs they once held about their identity, purpose, or appearance may no longer feel true. By strengthening these internal foundations, women create a deeper sense of continuity and self-trust—even as the external landscape evolves.

Each "self" plays a unique role in restoring confidence and vitality. Menopause calls for a deeper relationship with self. Self-worth reminds a woman she is valuable beyond roles or appearance. Self-respect helps her honor her changing needs without apology. Self-trust allows her to listen to her body and make choices with confidence. Self-reflection gives her space to grow, not just cope. Self-compassion softens the journey — offering grace instead of judgment, and kindness instead of criticism, as she reclaims her identity with strength and tenderness. Together, these "selves" don't just help women survive menopause—they help us rewrite the narrative and thrive in a powerful new chapter. It is the Foundation of Wholeness.

I've lived through every challenge and every twist and turn of these "selves." Each one tested me differently as I walked through my own transition. The path wasn't always clear. But eventually, I began embracing the small, steady practices that invited me back to myself:

journaling, quiet affirmations, and those tender moments in front of the mirror. "I am somebody and I am worthy." The unexpected gift in all of this is—the woman I met on the other side of that journey wasn't some polished version of who I used to be. She was someone I had never met before... not even in my most confident younger years. This "new me" carries a different kind of strength—grounded, intuitive, more forgiving with herself, and far less concerned with pleasing the world. Rebuilding those lost pieces didn't just return me to myself—It introduced me to someone more whole. That's the power of self-compassion, and if I could find her... so can you.

Conclusion

Menopause isn't the end of your vitality—It's the beginning of a reclamation. It's the moment when your many inner "selves," once quiet in the background, begin to rise and take the lead. Your self-image shifts—from external appearance to inner radiance. Your self-esteem uncouples from roles and resumes, returning to your inherent worth. Last but not least, your self-compassion becomes the soft, steady ground where you can finally breathe. This is the soul work of menopause. Not just surviving the symptoms—but reconnecting with the parts of you that were silenced, stretched thin, or forgotten altogether.

You are not fading.

You are unfolding.

You're not starting over.

You're finally meeting yourself.

Let this be your season to break free from doubt and step boldly into unapologetic self-confidence—rooted in every part of who you are, and blooming into who you're becoming. This is your time to reclaim your voice, your rhythm, and your worth. The woman emerging now is not a lesser version of who you once were—but a fuller expression of all she has lived, learned, and let go of. So yes, menopause is your invitation to break free from doubt and rise into something unapologetically powerful. The best part about this whole journey? You're just getting started. I know I am. "Beyond the Footprints of Menopause" is not just a title—it's a promise. A promise to honor every version of you: the self that doubted, the self that endured, the self that awakened, and the self that now stands whole.

Affirmation: *"When I look in the mirror, I see more than features. I see worth, wisdom, and a woman becoming. I am enough, just as I am—and I reflect beauty from the inside out."*

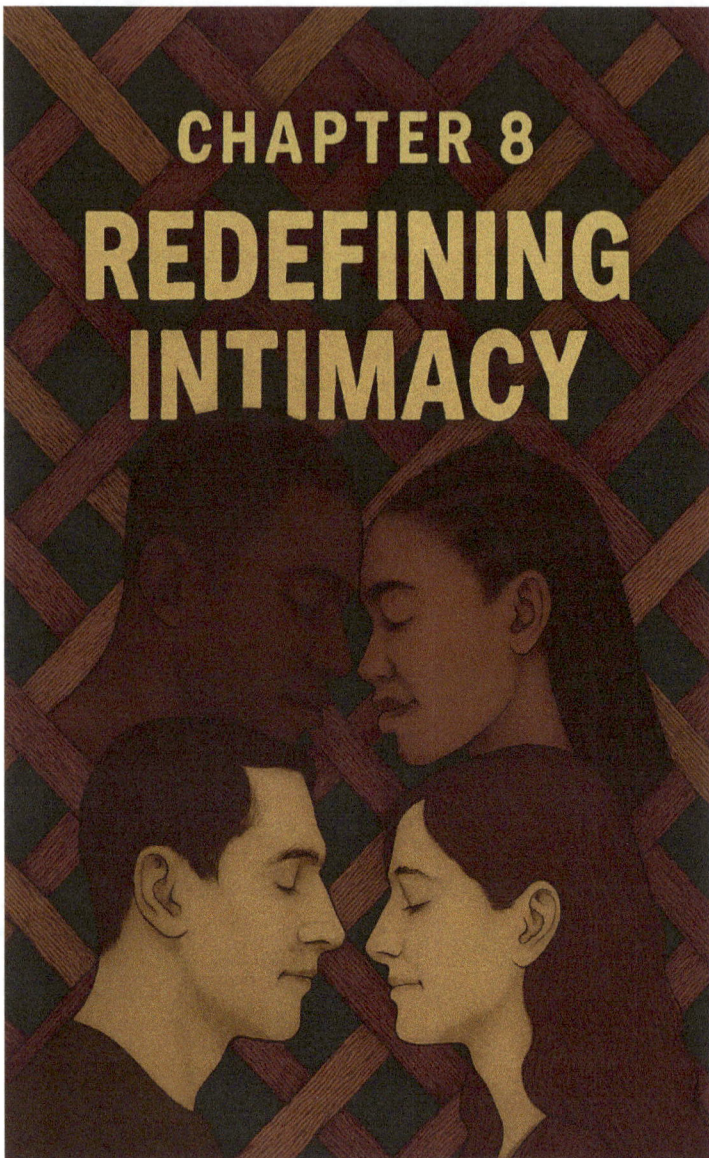

CHAPTER 8
REDEFINING INTIMACY

8 Redefining Intimacy: What Menopause Teaches Us About Love and Connection

The menopause era can profoundly shift a woman's inner world, and as that inner world changes, so can her connections with the people closest to her. It can affect her relationships with her husband, family, and close friends. Hormonal fluctuations may impact mood, energy, memory, libido, and the overall capacity to show up in the ways she's always known. It can create confusion or distance in relationships, especially if loved ones are unaware of what she's navigating. A partner might mistake withdrawal for disinterest, or family members might misread irritability as personal rather than physiological. Without open dialogue, misunderstandings can easily build, making an already challenging time feel even more isolating.

Yet menopause also offers a powerful opportunity for deeper connection. When a woman begins to understand and honor what she's going through, she can invite her loved ones into that awareness—helping them see that her symptoms are not the whole of who she is. With honest conversations, shared learning, and a shift in expectations, relationships can transform. This phase becomes a bridge—not a barrier—when those closest to you are willing to walk beside you with compassion, curiosity, and a bit more grace than usual. Because at its heart, this is not just about menopause; it's about growing together through one of life's most honest evolutions.

This chapter is about holding onto these relationships—and even deepening them—as you move through your menopause journey. It's about having honest conversations, setting healthy boundaries, and creating moments of joy and meaning with the people who matter the most.

Weathering the Storm Together: The Two of Us Through the Change

When a woman is going through the menopause journey, and the emotions are tagging along with her, they often tag onto her husband as well. Even though he may not experience the physical symptoms firsthand, he is very much on this journey too— walking beside his wife through a landscape neither of them fully expected. While she may be facing fatigue, mood shifts, or changes in libido, he's often left trying to understand what's happening and how to respond. The emotional climate of the relationship begins to shift—sometimes subtly, sometimes drastically—and it can leave both partners feeling disconnected. The husband's experience may be indirect, but it's real. Without clear communication or shared understanding, confusion and distance can quietly build.

Menopause doesn't just ask the woman to evolve; it invites the relationship to evolve, too. When both partners recognize that they're in this together, it opens the door to deeper empathy, mutual support, and even renewed intimacy. The goal is not to suffer in silence—it's to walk the path side by side with honesty, curiosity, and grace. Because the truth is, when a woman changes, the relationship changes— and so does the man who truly chooses to stay present through it all.

Talking Through the Tension: Communication That Connects, Not Collides

Open communication is the heartbeat of any strong relationship—whether a woman is navigating menopause or not. It's the thread that holds connection, trust, and emotional safety together. But let's be honest: for many couples, that thread can fray during the menopause transition. As a woman's internal world shifts, communication often becomes strained—not from a lack of love, but from a lack of understanding, space, and sometimes the right words to bridge the growing gap. There's no definitive research proving that the divorce rate is higher for couples during menopause, but there is research that reveals that menopause can place significant strain on the marriage.

When menopause enters a relationship, it often brings unspoken tension with it—because neither partner fully understands the ground shifting beneath them. During menopause, a woman may have mood swings, fatigue, memory lapses, or changes in libido, which can lead to misinterpretation and emotional distance.

The woman may retreat while the man feels shut out. When words finally surface, they are sometimes wrapped in frustration instead of understanding. This is why communication becomes not just important, but essential. Honest dialogue—grounded in compassion rather than blame—can shift the atmosphere from reactive to responsive. I experienced this strain in my own marriage, but things began to change when I realized that open communication was one of the keys to keeping the relationship strong.

As I mentioned, communication is the key—but it's not the only factor in holding a marriage together. Holding a marriage together during what some might describe as a storm takes more than words. It takes patience, empathy, adaptability, and a willingness to grow together, even when the path feels unfamiliar.

To connect instead of colliding, couples need a new communication rhythm—one that honors vulnerability, sets aside judgment, and replaces assumptions with curiosity. It's not about solving everything in one conversation but about building a safe space where both people can speak and be heard.

A meaningful conversation might begin with saying, "I'm struggling, and I don't fully understand it myself," can open more doors than silence or resentment ever could. Talking through the tension isn't always comfortable, but it's where intimacy is rebuilt—word by word, truth by truth, together.

From Frustration to Connection: How a Wife Can Shift the Tone

Lead with Emotional Clarity, Not Blame

Instead of saying, "You never understand how I feel!" try, I'm feeling overwhelmed, and I don't always know how to explain what's happening. This shifts the tone from accusation to vulnerability, inviting understanding rather than defensiveness.

Use "I" Statements to Express Needs

I need some quiet time after work to decompress, or I'd feel really supported if you could ask me how I'm doing more often. These statements are clear, gentle, and rooted in self-awareness; they help your partner know how to show up without feeling criticized. This one worked for me. Make sure you choose the correct tone. We have all heard it before—it's not only what you say, but how you say it is equally important. The tone of a woman's voice means everything to the person she is communicating with. Remember, you can say these words, but if the correct tone is not there, you may not get the right response back from your spouse. That awareness helped me feel more empowered instead of reactive. Over time, that softened the space between my husband and me. It reminded me that I was not just asking for understanding — I was also learning how to extend it. That made all the difference in the world.

Choose the Right Moment

Hard conversations don't land well when either partner is distracted, tired, or emotionally charged. Set intentional time aside for check-ins — perhaps over coffee or during a quiet walk — when both people can really be present. Timing is a tool, too. I learned this the hard way. For the longest time, I tried to bring up important conversations the moment they hit my heart. But over time, I noticed a pattern: when my husband was not in good headspace, those talks often went sideways or nowhere at all. Eventually, I realized it's okay to wait. It doesn't mean swallowing your truth; it means honoring the moment, so your message has space to land. It's not about walking on eggshells for weeks but about choosing calm over chaos when it really counts. Once I started being intentional with timing, I saw how much more connected and open our conversations became. I'm not saying you need to tiptoe around him for two weeks straight. But giving him space to mentally reset—before diving into heavy topics—can make a big difference in how he responds.

Name What's Changing Together

Start the conversation with- This stage of life is new for both of us. I don't always have the words for it, but I want us to learn together. What I need most is patience, understanding, and the space to share what I'm going through, even when I can't explain it perfectly. Your support doesn't have to come with all the answers—just being present makes all the difference. This will open up a shared experience.

When a wife includes her husband in the journey, it creates a partnership rather than separation.

Invite, Don't Demand

To get your partner to listen instead of becoming defensive, consider saying, Can we talk about how this phase is affecting us? Rather than, you never listen to me. The tone of invitation encourages a more open-hearted exchange. When you frame it as an invitation, the other person feels included rather than blamed. This shift lowers defensiveness and creates space for understanding instead of conflict. Small changes in wording can transform a difficult conversation into a bridge for connection. It's not about winning an argument, but about creating a safe place where both voices can be heard.

Use Gentle Metaphors

Sometimes emotions are hard to name directly. Saying things like, It feels like the ground is shifting under me lately or I'm carrying a lot of emotion that is weighing me down right now, paints a picture he can step into with empathy, even if he can't relate firsthand. It allows him to see the weight you're carrying without feeling blamed, and it opens the door for gentle questions or offers of support. Over time, these vivid images can help him understand your experience more deeply, making your conversations feel safer and more connected.

When I began applying these approaches, everything started to shift. Conversations felt less like battles and more like bridges, even on days when emotions ran high. I began to notice that when I approached my husband with calm, clarity, and better timing, he responded with more patience and presence. We weren't perfect, but we were reconnecting — slowly and steadily

Loving Through the Shift: How Men Can Stand Steady in Her Storm

Learn Before You React

When men are educated and understand what menopause is and how it affects a woman, physically, emotionally, and hormonally, it helps them take things less personally. When a husband educates himself, he can see mood swings or distance not as a rejection, but as part of what she's managing internally. A little understanding goes a long way in softening tension.

Listen Without Trying to Fix

Sometimes she just needs to be heard, not solved. A man can hold space by saying things like, "Do you want me to listen or help find a solution?" This shows emotional presence and honors her experience. By resisting the urge to immediately fix, he communicates that her feelings are valid and worthy of attention. Listening without jumping to solutions builds trust and deepens connection, creating a safe environment where vulnerability is welcomed rather than judged. Over time, this practice transforms everyday conversations into moments of true understanding and intimacy.

Check In, Don't Check Out

As communication patterns shift, it's tempting for the husband to pull away — but that's when his emotional availability matters most. Simple check-ins like, "How are you feeling today?" or "What can I do that would feel supportive right now?" can make her feel seen, heard, and valued.

Stay Open to Change

She's evolving, and the relationship will evolve too. That might mean rethinking intimacy, shifting responsibilities, or being okay with plans changing at the last minute. Flexibility and grace have become emotional superpowers here. For example, he might notice that she's more tired in the evenings and suggest switching date nights to earlier in the day, or taking on household tasks without being asked, so she has the space to recharge. Communicating openly: He could check in regularly with questions like, "How are you feeling about our routine lately?" or "Is there anything I can do differently to make things easier for you?" This keeps the dialogue flexible and collaborative. Supporting new self-care routines: If she starts a new exercise or mindfulness practice, he might join her occasionally or rearrange schedules so she can maintain it; this demonstrates adaptability and shared commitment to her well-being. These small adjustments show awareness, respect, and a willingness to adapt as life shifts and transforms.

His Self-Care Matters Too

Supporting someone through a transformation requires energy. It's easy for a man to become emotionally exhausted while supporting his wife through menopause, and without balance, he can experience burnout. Caring for himself is just as important as caring for her. He needs his outlets — friends to talk to, physical movement, hobbies that ground him — so he doesn't become emotionally depleted or resentful. Having his own outlet keeps him emotionally strong. Set healthy boundaries so you can offer support without depleting yourself. Even small moments of rest or personal time make a big difference. Communicate openly about your own needs and feelings. Process your feelings through personal reflection, journaling, or quiet activities that help you stay centered, rather than seeking guidance that might not fit your situation. Remember that self-care is not selfish—it's essential. Caring for yourself allows you to show up fully and compassionately for her.

Say the Hard Thing Kindly

If he feels hurt, confused, or distanced, he should name it gently. Instead of saying, "You're being unreasonable," he could say, "I notice this situation is really frustrating for you—how can I support you right now?" Instead of, "I don't understand why you're not interested," he could say, "I miss our closeness, and I want to understand how you're feeling so we can stay connected. "Instead of, "You're not keeping up with things like before," he could say, "I see things feel different lately—how can we adjust so it feels manageable for both of us?" Saying hard things kindly helps maintain connection and trust even when emotions are high. It allows her to hear the truth without feeling attacked, reducing defensiveness and opening space for honest dialogue. This approach strengthens the relationship by showing respect, empathy, and a willingness to understand her experience. Over time, it creates a pattern where both partners feel safe expressing needs and frustrations, turning potentially difficult conversations into opportunities for deeper intimacy and mutual support.

A New Fabric of Love

Menopause can tug at the fabric of a relationship, loosening the threads that once held it tightly together. But when couples choose to face the discomfort with openness, compassion, and curiosity, they begin weaving a new layer of closeness — one that embraces her transformation, his questions, and their shared strength. Their lives and emotions become like interwoven threads, creating a fabric that is different, yet stronger and more resilient.

Staying Close, Growing Stronger: Family, Friendship, and Menopause

The physical symptoms, mood changes, and emotional swings can quietly lead women to withdraw—choosing solitude over conversation or retreating into silence because it feels easier than explaining what's happening inside. But isolation during menopause can deepen feelings of loneliness, anxiety, and even depression. It can rob you of perspective, leaving you to carry burdens alone that were never meant to be yours in isolation. Menopause is often described as a deeply personal journey—but it was never meant to be a lonely one. While your body and mind navigate unfamiliar territory, the steady presence of family and friends can become an anchor and a reminder that you're still surrounded by love, history, and connection.

That's why it's so important to stay intentional about keeping those bonds alive. Whether it's a quick phone call, a shared cup of tea, or a heartfelt talk about how you're really feeling, these simple connections can become powerful lifelines. Now is the perfect time to create new memories and simple traditions that spark joy. Plan casual brunches, game nights, or walks in the park with a trusted friend. Try new experiences together—whether it's a pottery class, a weekend getaway, or a shared playlist of songs that make you want to dance in your kitchen. These don't have to be grand gestures: often, it's the small, silly, everyday moments that leave the deepest imprint. Cultivating

joy isn't about ignoring what's hard—it's about choosing to make space for what uplifts you, alongside those who remind you how good it feels to smile, laugh, and truly live.

Joy and Laughter Is Not a Luxury—It's Medicine

Joy is one of the most underrated strengths for emotional resilience during menopause. Shared laughter has a way of dissolving tension, softening heavy days, and reminding you that life—even in its most challenging seasons—still holds moments worth celebrating. Taking time to laugh with family and friends isn't trivial—it's a lifeline. These moments of levity provide emotional release, strengthen bonds, and bring balance to a journey that can often feel overwhelming. The people who have walked beside you through life's ups and downs can offer comfort, perspective, and even laughter when you need it the most.

Menopause may change how you show up in the world, but it doesn't have to separate you from the hearts that have shaped your story. This season offers a beautiful opportunity to grow closer and stronger—together. Staying connected is not a luxury—it's a form of emotional self-care, a lifeline that reminds you you're still loved, valued, and seen, even when you don't feel like yourself.

There's Healing Power in Community.

There's healing power in the community, especially during a life shift as complex and personal as menopause. In the midst of emotional swings, physical changes, and moments of deep self-doubt, knowing you're not alone can be a lifeline. Talking with other women who truly understand what you're going through — not because they read about it, but because they're living it too — can ease the isolation and validate your experience. Community offers more than just support; it provides perspective, encouragement, and often, laughter in the moments that feel the heaviest. When we come together and share openly, we begin to see that our struggles are not signs of weakness but threads in a collective story of strength and resilience.

When They Don't Understand: Standing Strong in the Face of Misunderstanding

One of the hardest parts of menopause is not just managing your symptoms, but it also involves navigating the reactions of people who don't understand what you're going through. Well-meaning loved ones might dismiss your experience with comments like, "It's just a phase," or "everyone goes through it—you'll be fine." Others may pull away emotionally, unsure of how to support you, or be uncomfortable with the changes that they have witnessed.

These moments can sting, making you feel unseen or invalidated. But it's important to remember that not everyone will grasp the depth of this transition—and their misunderstanding often says more about their discomfort or lack of awareness than it does about your worth or what you deserve. This is where compassionate, clear boundaries become essential. You have every right to protect your emotional space and energy without guilt. That might mean calmly addressing hurtful remarks, explaining what you need in the moment or choosing to step away from conversations that drain you.

Setting boundaries doesn't mean cutting people out; it means teaching others how to treat you with respect and care during this sensitive season. Give yourself permission to prioritize your peace and surround yourself with people who honor your journey, even if it means finding that support in new places. You are allowed to expect kindness and understanding—and to walk away from anything that makes your healing harder.

Key Lessons Learned and Wisdom to Carry Forward

Throughout this chapter, we explored how menopause often brings new challenges to intimacy in romantic relationships and relationships with family and friends. Changes in libido, physical discomfort, body image struggles, and emotional fluctuations can test even the strongest partnerships. Yet within these challenges emerges an opportunity for a deeper connection. When we choose to communicate openly with our partners, express not just our needs but also our fears and insecurities, we create space for honest, tender moments of understanding. True intimacy is not about perfection; it's about growing together, embracing each other's humanity, and nurturing emotional closeness.

We discussed how friendships and family bonds can either be strengthened or strained during this time. Menopause often requires a new kind of support — one rooted in patience, humor, and compassion. Some people in your life may not fully understand what you're experiencing, and that's okay. Part of this journey is learning to release unrealistic expectations and instead focus your energy on those who choose to stand beside you with kindness and grace. Building new connections with women going through similar experiences can offer unexpected healing, reminding you that sisterhood is one of the most powerful antidotes to isolation.

Menopause offers a key opportunity to reconsider and redefine intimacy in a way that aligns with who you are now. It might mean a spontaneous hug from your child, a long walk with a dear friend, or a playful moment of laughter with your husband. It could be the quiet peace of sitting in your own company, reconnecting with yourself in a way you never allowed before. This season invites you to stop measuring intimacy by the old standards and instead embrace the richness of connection in all its newest forms — physical, emotional, and spiritual.

We touched on how lighthearted moments, and shared experiences can be powerful tools for resilience. In the heaviness of midlife transitions, joy and laughter are not distractions but necessities. Creating space for fun, simplicity, and spontaneous connection offers balance and reminds you that menopause, while often challenging, is also a chapter of life that holds beauty, growth, and opportunities for meaningful connection.

Conclusion

As we close this chapter, it's important to pause and reflect on the beautiful — and sometimes complicated ways menopause reshapes how we experience love, connection, and intimacy. This season of life invites us to confront not only the physical changes within our bodies but also the shifts within our relationships. Menopause teaches us that intimacy is not solely about physical closeness — it is about emotional presence, vulnerability, and a willingness to meet one another exactly where we are.

As you step away from this chapter, carry this truth with you: Menopause does not mark the end of love, desire, or meaningful relationships. It is an invitation to deepen, to soften, and to rediscover connection in ways you might not have explored before. It asks you to be brave enough to express your needs, open enough to receive support, and wise enough to release what no longer serves you.

This chapter of life — and this chapter of your book — is a reminder that intimacy isn't a fixed destination. It evolves with you. And as you continue through this journey, may you surround yourself with people who honor your heart, cherish your honesty, and walk with you as you redefine what love and connection look like in this powerful, unapologetic season of life.

Affirmation: *"As I change, so does the way I love, connect, and let others in. I honor this season as an invitation to deepen intimacy—with myself and with those who truly see me. I am worthy of love that grows, communication that heals, and connection that meets me where I am now."*

CHAPTER 9
Embracing The Best Version of You

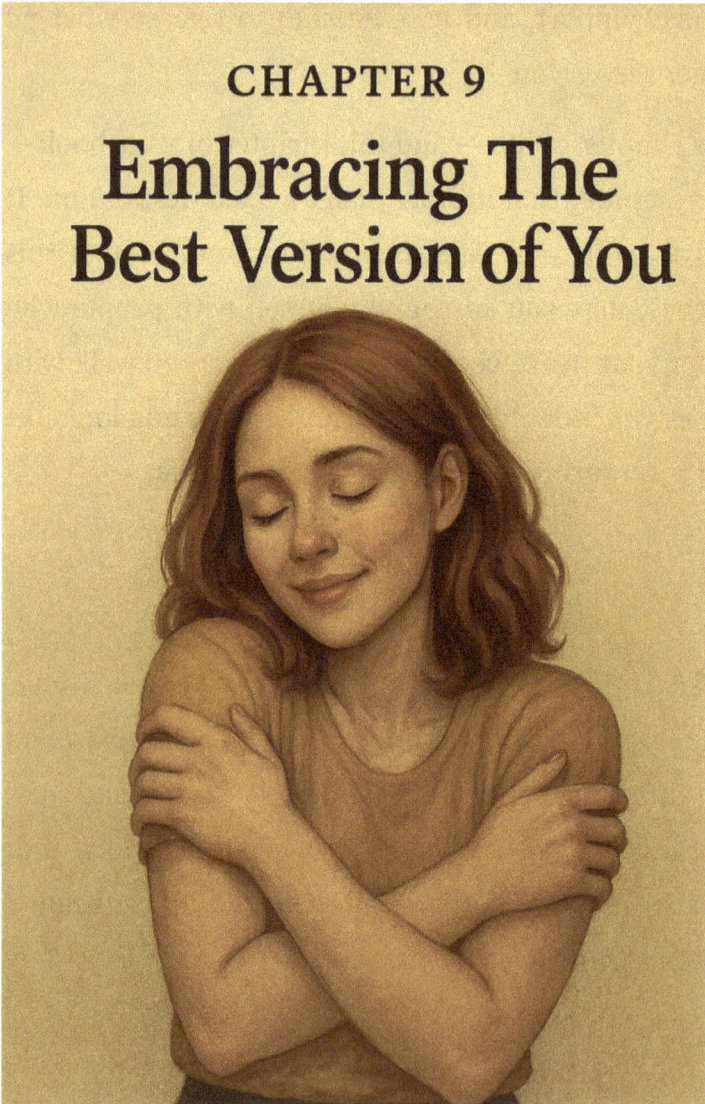

9 Embracing the Best Version of You: The Here and Now

This chapter begins with a shift in perspective: moving beyond longing for the past to embracing who you are today. Here, you'll explore how your experiences and wisdom have shaped you, and how you can step into this stage of life with confidence, authenticity, and a presence that reflects your true self. You'll discover ways to nurture your inner beauty, radiate self-assurance, and fully own the remarkable woman you have become today.

As we get older, it's normal to think back to when our skin felt firmer, our jeans zipped up more easily, let's just say our jeans now are getting more cozy with us, and our hair had that perfect bounce. We remember the strength and spark we once had and occasionally yearn for its return. Maybe you've seen someone rock an outfit and thought, 'I want that too! —only to realize it doesn't feel quite the same on you. At times, many of us still try to hold on to that younger version of ourselves, even if it's just a little.

The Challenges of Embracing Who We Once Were

Trying to hold onto a former version of ourselves can create a subtle emotional conflict between who we were and who we have become. The past may feel safer or more familiar, especially when facing new physical, emotional, or relational changes. We might cling to old routines, past appearances, or long-held identities that once defined us, believing they hold the key to confidence or vitality. But this resistance to change can lead to frustration, sadness, or self-doubt, especially when we measure our present against an outdated standard. The challenge lies in trying to recreate something that no longer fits while simultaneously ignoring the wisdom and growth we've gained.

There's also the danger of romanticizing our past selves, overlooking the nuance of what we actually lived through. When we embrace only the highlight reel of who we used to be, we may unintentionally minimize the depth of our current season. The truth is that transformation, especially through menopause, is not about loss; it's about evolution. When we attempt to reinhabit an earlier version of ourselves, we risk delaying the emotional and spiritual expansion that this stage offers. Instead of chasing old footsteps, the path forward asks us to create new footsteps, grounded in authenticity, compassion, and the courage to evolve.

I've lived through this chapter, the one where we try to anchor ourselves to the past, believing that if we hold on tightly enough, we can preserve what once was. Many of us pass through this phase, quietly mourning the version of ourselves we've outgrown. But it truly is just that, a phase. We were never meant to stay stuck there. Life is too broad, too layered, and too rich to be constrained by old expectations. The desire to cling to what we often call "fading youth" isn't really about age; it's about the emotions, the vitality, and the freedom we associate with that time. But what people refer to as fading youth during menopause is actually the fear of becoming invisible, the grief over what's shifting, and the uncertainty of who we are becoming.

While it's easy to romanticize what it once was, the present offers its own unique power, purpose, and beauty. I know personally that feeling of longing, the moments of self-doubt, and the search for my place in a culture that elevates youth above everything. But I've also learned that youthfulness doesn't vanish; it simply evolves. It grows quieter, deeper, and more intentional. Through menopause, I've learned that my worth isn't defined by who I was when I was younger. Instead, this phase reminds me that I'm still growing, evolving, and stepping into a fuller, more vibrant version of myself. I honor my journey—not by ignoring the changes, but by seeing them as evidence that I'm still becoming. Menopause is not a loss; it's an opportunity to reconnect with the vitality and potential that has always been within you.

The Truth About Fading Youth

The phrase "fading youth" is a literary and cultural expression rather than a formal technical term. It originates from the general idea of youth being temporary, emphasizing the natural passage of time and the visible or felt changes in the body, energy, and appearance as people age. Writers, poets, and social commentators often use it to evoke nostalgia, loss, or the societal obsession with youthfulness. In a society that glorifies youth, menopause can feel like a marker of fading youth, a sign that you're moving out of the culturally prized season. Women may notice changes in physical appearance, skin texture, hair thinning, weight shifts, the presence of lines and wrinkles, and no longer being able to conceive. This can trigger unexpected feelings of loss. When menopause is associated with fading youth, it's really about confronting and redefining what aging means as a woman—and reclaiming that narrative on your own terms.

This is how I look at fading youth since I have learned how to thrive through menopause. Instead of saying "fading youth," I like to look at it as ripening years, the closing of one chapter and the awakening of another. Fading youth doesn't mean losing value; it means moving into a new stage of life where wisdom, confidence, and self-awareness take center stage. Fading youth reminds us that life is a journey of transformation, giving us the chance to define beauty, purpose, and fulfillment on our own terms. As we get older, it opens the door to discovering strengths, passions, and joys that only come with experience and growth. Fading youth doesn't mean fading worth, beauty, or significance. Many women find that post-menopause becomes their most powerful, liberated season yet—unburdened by societal expectations tied to youth.

Beyond Society's Standards: Freedom from External Expectations

When women are no longer bound by societal pressures to look or behave a certain way, women often find a new sense of authenticity and self-expression. With age comes rich experience, emotional intelligence, and clarity. The fading of youth makes space for deeper insight and intuitive power. Beauty becomes less about appearance and more about presence, vitality, and emotional resonance. It's a shift from surface to soul. Many women stop performing roles for others and begin living for themselves—choosing what truly nourishes them physically, emotionally, and spiritually. The fading of youth can symbolize the shedding of outdated identities, making room for transformation, creativity, and purpose. The fading of youth makes space for deeper insight and intuitive power.

Embracing the Body's Evolution

Our bodies are constantly changing, and menopause marks a significant chapter in that ongoing evolution. Embracing these changes means seeing them not as losses, but as signs of growth, resilience, and transformation. Every curve, line, and shift tells the story of the life you've lived and the wisdom you've gained. By honoring your body's evolution, you step into a deeper sense of self-acceptance, confidence, and vitality—recognizing that beauty and strength are not fixed in youth but continue to flourish at every stage of life. Instead of resisting change, women can learn to honor their bodies as wise, adaptive, and worthy—just as they are.

The Beauty of Becoming: Letting Go of Yesterday, Living Fully Today

As you journey through menopause, one of the quiet griefs many women carry is the sense of losing the version of beauty they once knew. But holding on to that image keeps you anchored in a past that no longer serves the woman you are becoming. The truth is that beauty isn't something you lose; it's something that evolves. It softens, deepens, and begins to live in places the world can't always see, in your kindness, your wisdom, your resilience, and the way you show up fully in your life, unfiltered and unafraid.

To overcome the pull of the past, you must consciously redefine what beauty means to you, on your own terms. Begin by noticing the qualities in yourself that have nothing to do with appearance but everything to do with presence: the warmth of your laugh, the steady way you comfort others, the courage it takes to face uncertainty. Let yourself grieve what's changing, but don't stay there. Create new rituals that celebrate this chapter of your life: wear colors that lift your spirit, speak words to yourself you would offer a dear friend. Beauty now lives in your authenticity, in your capacity for joy, and in the light you bring into every room you enter. When you begin to see yourself through this lens, you will realize you have not lost beauty at all; you have simply uncovered its truest form. When you begin to see yourself through this lens, you'll carry a confidence and radiance that others can't help but notice, revealing the true beauty within you.

Create Rituals that Honor the Present

One of the most healing things you can do during menopause is to create simple, intentional rituals that anchor you in the here and now. It's easy to get caught up in mourning what's behind you or worrying about what's ahead, but peace is always found in the present moment. Whether it's lighting a candle before bed, enjoying a slow cup of tea in the quiet morning hours, or taking a few minutes to stretch and breathe deeply at sunset, these small acts of presence are sacred. They remind you that your life is still unfolding, still sacred, and still yours to shape, no matter what season you're in.

These rituals don't have to be elaborate. In fact, the simpler, the better. Journaling a single sentence about what you're grateful for, placing fresh flowers on your table, or standing barefoot in the grass can all become meaningful ways to reconnect with yourself. The key is to be fully present when you do them, to pause, notice and feel. In honoring these small moments, you remind yourself that beauty isn't just found in the milestones of youth, but in the quiet, ordinary, everyday experiences that nurture your soul. Through rituals, you root yourself in the truth that life remains beautiful, meaningful, and worthy, right here, and right now.

Dress for the You of Today

The way you present yourself to the world is a reflection of how you feel inside, and menopause is the perfect time to release old ideas about how you should look and instead dress in a way that honors who you are right now. So often, women hold onto clothes or styles that belong to a younger version of themselves, out of nostalgia or a quiet fear of change. But true confidence comes when you dress in a way that aligns with the woman you have become, not the one you used to be. Choose colors, fabrics, and silhouettes that feel good on your skin, flatter your shape as it is today, and this will make you feel seen and beautiful in your own eyes.

Style yourself in clothes that reflect who you are now, not in competition with your past self or anyone else, but with confidence and authenticity. Wear what makes you feel vibrant, powerful, and at ease. Dressing for the you of today is a form of self-respect and self-celebration. It says, This is who I am now, and I deserve to feel good in my own skin. Wearing what makes you feel confident doesn't just change how others perceive you; it changes how you move through life. This was another one of those challenging moments for me. I held onto so many clothes from my past—pieces I kept wearing because they represented the youthful version of me. But one day, something shifted. I began to wake up to the truth: I'm not that person anymore. I've grown. I'm more resilient, more grounded. And those clothes? They didn't fit who I've become. I refreshed my wardrobe—not to fit someone else's idea of what I should wear, but to showcase my personality and style now. I began to feel a sense of relief and freedom once I realized those clothes no longer fit the new me.

Celebrate Your Body for What It Can Still Do

It's easy to focus on what's changed in your body during menopause, the areas that ache a little more, the stamina that isn't quite what it was, or the softness in places that once felt firm. But what if you shift your attention to everything your body still does for you every single day? This body has carried you through joy and heartbreak, through sleepless nights and radiant mornings. It wakes up each day, breathes life into your moments, and allows you to laugh, dance, hug, and create. There is deep, undeniable beauty in a body that endures, adapts, and continues to serve you, no matter how it evolves.

Rather than measure your worth by a number on a scale or a reflection in the mirror, begin celebrating your body for its strength, its resilience, and its quiet, everyday miracles. Honor your legs for the miles they have walked, your hands for the love they have given, your heart for the burdens it carried and the joys that it welcomed. Every wrinkle, scar, and stretch mark tells a story of a life fully lived. When you shift your focus from what's been lost to what remains, and what is still possible, you reconnect with a sense of gratitude and reverence for the incredible vessel that has carried you this far and will continue to carry you into your next beautiful chapter. Dance in the kitchen. Stretch with intention. Fuel it with kindness. The body may change, but it's still a vessel of strength, love, and sacred power.

Engage Your Curiosity

Curiosity is not just for the young; it is the inner flame that keeps us alive, alert, and ever evolving. As we grow older, our perspective expands, allowing us to explore with greater intention and depth. Learning a new skill or diving into a creative project is not about keeping up; it is about reconnecting with the pieces of ourselves we may have tucked away. That painting class you never tried, the book you wanted to write, the garden you imagined is still waiting, and you can bring more wisdom and richness to it now than ever before. Your curiosity has seasoned over time, like a vintage wine, aged, complex, and more satisfying with every sip.

In this season of life, every moment can be an act of discovery. When you embrace curiosity, you shake loose the outdated idea that aging is synonymous with limitation. Instead, you transform it into an invitation to pursue wonder, to ask what if, and to say yes to the unfamiliar. Whether it is cooking with bold new spices, studying something totally outside your field, or exploring stories you've never told, let your curiosity guide you into new dimensions of joy and fulfillment. There is no age limit to curiosity; it is the heartbeat of reinvention, and it can lead you boldly into a life that is richer, more vibrant, and wholly yours.

In creating my menopause program and writing *Beyond the Footprints of Menopause*, I have embodied the very spirit of curiosity and reinvention, and I encourage others to do the same. What began as a whisper of possibility grew into a calling and a creative pursuit fueled by my own experiences, questions, and reflections. I dove into research, explored symbolism and crafted rituals that spoke to the emotional shifts women face in this season. Through every landing page, every certificate, every word written, I have rediscovered passions that once sat dormant. This work is not just professional, it is personal. It is proof that curiosity doesn't fade; it evolves. By nurturing my curiosity, I have built a path for others to walk more boldly into their own transformation.

Speak Kindly to Yourself

Speaking kindly to yourself is not just about affirmations; it is about rewriting the internal narrative that has too often been shaped by comparison, criticism, and unrealistic expectations. In a world that praises youth and sometimes perfection, it takes courage to look in the mirror and offer yourself compassion. Every wrinkle, every shift, every season of change holds stories of strength. When we soften our tone inwardly, we begin to heal the harshness we've carried. Self-kindness is a practice, a gentle unfolding, and a daily invitation to treat ourselves with the same grace we extend to others. Kindness to self becomes especially powerful during transitions like menopause, when emotions, identity, and relationships may feel unsettled. In this space, your inner voice can either uplift or undo you. Choosing kindness is not a weakness; it is self-respect. It is speaking words that soothe rather than shame, celebrating resilience rather than mourning change. The more gently we speak to ourselves, the more confidently we show up for life, for love, and for our purpose. Through self-kindness, we rediscover a deeper version of self-worth, one not rooted in what we used to be, but in the wisdom of who we are now. Release the inner critic. Replace those negative echoes with:

I honor the woman I am becoming.

I am proud of how far I've come.

I choose to celebrate my strengths and growth.

I am worthy of joy, love, and abundance.

I embrace my journey and all that it teaches me.

I am evolving into my best self every day.

I trust myself and my decisions.

I deserve to shine and be fully seen.

Look in the mirror, speak it, and claim it. Your words create your inner landscape. This is embracing the best version of you.

Unapologetically Yourself

To be unapologetically yourself means dropping the need for external validation and embracing who you are with radical honesty and pride. It's the permission to be bold in your truth, even when it doesn't fit into neat societal molds. It's the moment you stop shrinking to make others comfortable, and instead take up space with your stories, your voice, and your unique perspective. Especially during seasons of transformation, like menopause, there's power in shedding roles that no longer serve you and stepping into authenticity without apology. You don't have to justify your joy, your boundaries, your softness, or your strength. You get to be whole, and you get to be seen. Living unapologetically also means honoring your evolution. You are allowed to change your mind, grow past old expectations, and realign with who you've become. It's not defiance, it is freedom. When you show up fully as yourself, you permit others to do the same. Your presence becomes a quiet revolution and a daily act of empowerment. This is not about being loud for the sake of noise; it's about being rooted in truth, guided by courage, and fueled by self-respect. Being unapologetically you is not a destination; it is a practice, and it is the path toward living a life that feels deeply aligned and fiercely authentic.

Here and Now

The "here and now" is where your life unfolds—not in the regrets of yesterday or the uncertainties of tomorrow, but in this very moment. It's easy to get caught in the tides of what used to be or what might come next, but the true power lies in anchoring yourself right now. Every breath, every choice, every interaction offers a chance to connect with your values, your joy, and your aliveness. It's not about rushing through your days; it is about noticing them. The warmth of sunlight through your window, the quiet stirrings of intuition, the tiny victories you almost forgot to celebrate—all of it matters. When we choose presence, we find peace, and in that peace, there is strength.

Being grounded in the here and now is a form of mental clarity. It is the recognition that you are no longer chasing an idealized version of yourself; You are living as your truest self. This moment is rich with everything you've lived and everything you are becoming. When you show up fully, you reclaim your time, your energy, and your truth; and from that place, the journey becomes less about fixing and more about flourishing. The here and now is not just a pause; it's your stage, your sanctuary, your invitation to live well.

Living in the present as we age is truly an act of grace, and a mindset shift that can restore joy and freedom. Instead of chasing what once was, celebrate what is becoming. Beauty can be radiant in your eyes, wisdom in your words, or serenity in your presence.

Conclusion

While your youth is giving way to a new, vibrant phase, it makes room for a new chapter rich with wisdom, freedom, self-assurance, and deeper purpose. We can't rewind time. What we can do is shift our focus. Instead of clinging to the past, we can choose to live in the present, embracing the beautiful, powerful version of ourselves today. It is time to embrace *The Best Version of You*. When we shift our focus to looking and feeling our best at this moment, at this stage of life, we begin

to grieve less over what was and celebrate more of what still is. Youthfulness doesn't disappear; it simply transforms. We can carry it gracefully into our current season without pretending to be a version of ourselves that no longer fits.

We are not walking in the shadows of who we once were. We are stepping boldly into the light of who we are becoming. Stepping beyond the footprints of menopause means letting go of what no longer serves you and welcoming the new version of yourself. The best is not behind us. It is blooming right here and right now.

Affirmation: *"I release the echoes of who I was and stand fully in the grace of who I am. My power lives in the present, not in the past."*

CHAPTER 10
Too Old For What?

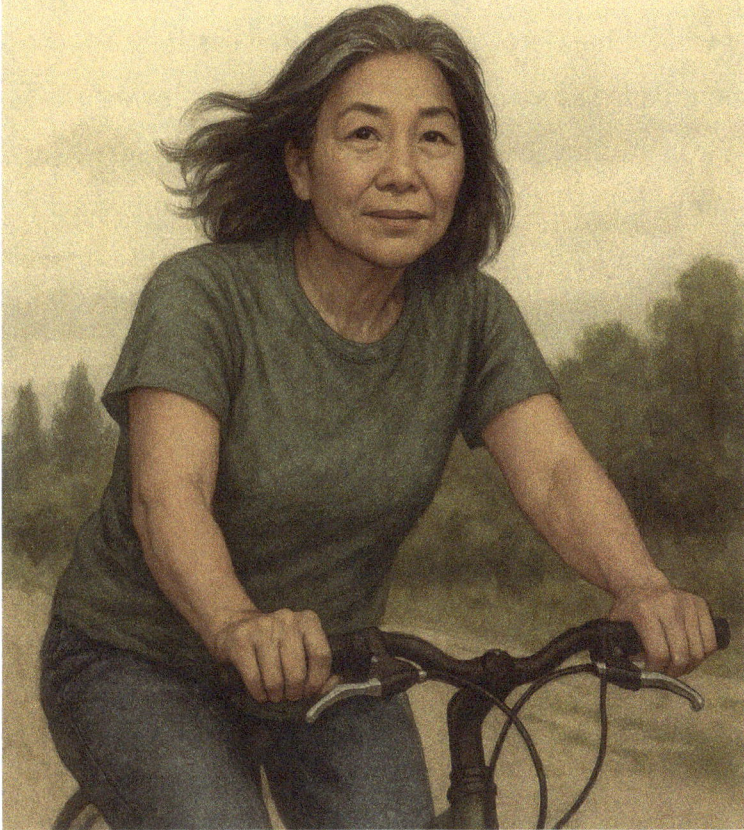

10 Too Old for What? To stop becoming? Not a chance

This chapter is all about shedding light on the myths that have shaped how we see aging and menopause, because when we know better, we live better. For far too long, society has boxed women into narrow ideas of what it means to grow older, often casting menopause as an endpoint rather than a powerful new beginning. These myths create unnecessary fear, shame, and limitation, convincing many women that their best years are behind them. In truth, the menopause journey can be far richer and more hopeful. By challenging these misconceptions, we reclaim our stories, rediscover our worth, and open the doors to possibilities that may have once seemed out of reach.

There's a quiet yet relentless message that echoes through our culture: that a woman's worth is tethered to her youth, her smooth skin, and how closely she can cling to the image of the girl she once was. Magazines, movies, ads, even casual conversations remind us in subtle — and sometimes not-so-subtle — ways that once menopause arrives, we're supposed to fade into the background, invisible, irrelevant, and unattractive. The menopausal years are not too old for adventure, passion, bold lipstick, or chasing our dreams.

Breaking Free from Society's Age Expectations

As we reach certain milestones in life, it's all too common to hear — or even believe — that we're "too old" for this or that. Society, with its relentless focus on youth, often sends messages that once you hit a certain age, your opportunities shrink, your dreams become less valid, and your time for growth or change is over.

Breaking free from society's age expectations means rejecting the narrow, often limiting beliefs about what women "should" or "should not" do as they grow older. For decades, cultural messages have told us that aging equals decline, invisibility, or a fading of relevance — especially for women. These expectations can create invisible walls, convincing many to shrink themselves, silence their dreams, or accept less than they deserve. However, the truth is these societal rules are just stories — stories that we have the power to rewrite. When women challenge these outdated norms, they reclaim their freedom to live boldly, pursue passions, and define their own versions of success and happiness.

This liberation is both a personal and collective journey. On a personal level, it requires mindfulness to recognize when we are internalizing limiting beliefs and courage to challenge them head-on. It also means surrounding ourselves with people and messages that uplift and affirm our worth at every age. Collectively, when more women break free and visibly live outside these age-related boxes, they shatter stereotypes and open doors for others to do the same. Breaking free from society's age expectations is an act of rebellion and self-love that transforms not only individual lives but the cultural narrative around aging itself.

Whether it's switching careers, learning something new, starting a new relationship, or simply embracing a new adventure, the assumption that age is a barrier can be discouraging and limiting. These beliefs are deeply ingrained, fueled by stereotypes and cultural expectations that tell us to slow down, step back, or settle for less.

But here's the truth that too few voices remind us of: Age is not a stop sign—it's a green light, inviting you to move forward, embrace new possibilities, and step boldly into what's next. Each year lays another stone beneath your feet, lifting you into a new perspective, a deeper purpose, and a strength you didn't know you had. The idea that we are "too old" to become more, to try new things, or to reinvent ourselves is simply a myth. Every decade of life brings unique gifts, wisdom, and opportunities to expand who we are. The barriers we imagine are often just fears dressed up as facts. Breaking free from these outdated beliefs is the first step toward embracing a life that is vibrant, purposeful, and endlessly evolving — regardless of the number attached to your birthday.

Flipping the Script on Age: No Shade, Just Truth

This world is so focused on youth and beauty, and some younger generations feel that when women get older, their lives are over. Wake up, young people—

we are so different from the grandmothers back in the day. This is not to disrespect the women who came before us, because each generation has paved the way for us to become who we are today. They laid the foundation and faced limitations we no longer have. We honor them by living fully. We are a new generation that is thriving more than ever. No shade, just truth. Aging isn't about slowing down or fading out; it's about moving forward with strength, wisdom, and undeniable grace.

Let's be real — back in the day, the idea of a woman over 50 skydiving? Unheard of. But today, we're flipping the script. This generation of women isn't slowing down; we're leaping forward, literally and figuratively. Just like the younger crowd, we're out here proving we can do just about anything. This generation of menopausal women is redefining what this season of life looks like. We're not confined to rocking chairs — we're rising, thriving, and stepping boldly into new possibilities.

So again, I say — too old for what? Too old to start over? Too old to fall in love with yourself? Too old to wear what makes you feel powerful? Too old to build something new, travel, reset, speak up, say no, say yes, or burn it all down and rebuild? Who decided that there's an expiration date on being extraordinary? Sure, we adapt as we grow older, but that doesn't mean we stop growing, dreaming, or daring. Get ready to let go of society's old rules. The only permission you need is your own.

Why society clings so tightly to youth

When you turn on your television, everything is about youth. Everyone wants to look 50 years younger than their age — well, maybe not quite. When you look in the mirror as you age, what do you see? Sometimes we don't even see ourselves; we have an image of what society thinks we should look like.

Society often equates youth with outward appearance, focusing on smooth skin and slender frames instead of the energy, curiosity, and vitality that truly define it. But youth isn't just about how you look — it's also about how you live, think, and feel. Why limit it to surface-level traits when its essence runs so much deeper? It's time we start recognizing the inner youth that shows up in resilience, joy, and the courage to keep growing.

Society often pushes the idea that we're no longer valuable as we age. The real challenge is that when we start internalizing those messages—especially the media's obsession with staying young—our minds can take over, influencing how we think, feel, and respond.

Here's the truth: our worth isn't defined by how young we look — it's grounded in how deeply we've lived. When we start to shift our focus inward, we reclaim the power to see ourselves through a lens of purpose, not pressure. Every wrinkle, every story, every breakthrough becomes a reminder that we're still becoming.

Society often sends the message that our value fades with age — but the real challenge is what happens in our own minds. When we constantly see youth glorified in the media, it can lead us to question our worth, and that self-doubt begins to shape how we think, feel, and respond. But we have the power to rewrite that narrative.

To Age with Purpose

To age with purpose means embracing each new chapter of life with intention, clarity, and a deep commitment to living fully. It's about recognizing that growing older is not about slowing down or stepping aside but about stepping into a richer version of yourself. Purpose gives life direction and fuels passion, no matter your age. When you age with purpose, you become more selective about where you invest your time, energy, and heart — choosing what truly matters to you and letting go of what doesn't. It's a conscious decision to live aligned with your values, dreams, and the legacy you want to leave behind. Only through aging do we gain the kind of wisdom that makes this possible. This is exactly why we can guide the younger generation, it allows us to pass real wisdom down—to offer not just advice, but experience, perspective, and strength. By sharing our wisdom and experiences, we can help younger generations uncover their strengths and walk confidently in their true purpose. A purposeful life in midlife and beyond is a powerful antidote to the stereotypes and doubts that often accompany aging. It invites you to explore new possibilities, deepen existing passions, and create meaningful connections that nourish your soul. Aging with purpose is not about fitting into anyone else's expectations; it's about honoring your unique journey and the wisdom you've gained along the way. When you move through life with this clarity, every day becomes an opportunity to make a difference — for yourself and for others — and to thrive in ways you might never have imagined.

Reclaiming Your Identity Beyond Menopause

Menopause often marks a significant turning point in a woman's life — not just physically, but emotionally and spiritually. For many, it brings a chance to step back and reflect on who they are beyond the roles they've played for years — whether as a mother, wife, or professional. It's a moment to reclaim identity that may have been overshadowed by caregiving responsibilities or societal expectations. Reclaiming your identity beyond menopause means reconnecting with your passions, values, and desires on your own terms. It's about rediscovering what truly lights you up and giving yourself permission to evolve into the fullest version of yourself, free from the constraints of how others expect you to show up.

This process isn't always easy — it requires honesty, patience, and sometimes grieving what has passed, so you can fully embrace what's next. But it's also deeply liberating. As you peel back layers of conditioned beliefs and outdated self-images, you begin to uncover the vibrant, authentic woman waiting to be expressed. Menopause can be a powerful catalyst for transformation, inviting you to create a new narrative rooted in self-awareness and self-love. By reclaiming your identity, you not only honor your journey but also set an inspiring example for other women to embrace their own unique paths beyond this life stage.

Living with Intention: Setting New Goals and Priorities

Living with intention means choosing how you spend your time, energy, and resources in a way that aligns deeply with what matters most to you. As you move through menopause and beyond, it's natural for priorities to shift, and this is a perfect opportunity to reassess your goals with fresh eyes. Instead of moving through life on autopilot or out of obligation, living intentionally invites you to be deliberate — whether that's nurturing your health, pursuing a new passion, strengthening relationships, or giving back to your community. Setting clear, meaningful goals rooted in your values gives you direction and motivation, turning each day into a purposeful step forward.

This intentional approach also means learning to say no to things that no longer serve your well-being or your vision for life. It's about creating space for what truly nourishes you and letting go of guilt around boundaries. When you focus on priorities that uplift and inspire you, you cultivate a sense of fulfillment that radiates into every area of your life. Living with intention transforms midlife from a time of loss or limitation into a powerful season of growth, creativity, and joy — because you are choosing to make this chapter one of your most vibrant yet.

The Power of Connection: Building Supportive Communities

The power of connection is undeniable, especially as we navigate the changes and challenges that come with menopause and midlife. Building supportive communities creates a space where women can share their experiences, celebrate their victories, and find comfort during difficult moments. These connections remind us that we are not alone in our journey and that our stories, struggles, and triumphs are part of a greater collective. A strong community offers encouragement, accountability, and a safe haven where authenticity is welcomed and valued. It is within these circles that healing accelerates and resilience grows, as we draw strength from one another's wisdom and compassion.

Supportive communities also inspire growth by exposing us to diverse perspectives and fresh ideas.

When women come together with openness and trust, they create fertile ground for learning, empowerment, and transformation. Through shared vulnerability and mutual respect, these connections spark creativity, ignite passion, and motivate us to reach beyond what we thought possible. Building and nurturing these relationships not only enriches our own lives but sets a powerful example for others to follow, weaving a network of women who uplift and propel each other toward greater fulfillment and purpose.

The Power of Lifelong Growth and Adaptability

The world is constantly changing, and by staying open to new ideas, technologies, and perspectives, we keep ourselves engaged and adaptable. Whether it's picking up a new skill, exploring a hobby, or simply staying informed about the things that interest you, continuous growth helps you stay connected to the world around you. Relevance isn't about trying to be someone you're not—it's about evolving authentically, bringing your unique experience and wisdom to the table while embracing what's new and exciting without losing sight of who we are.

Never Too Old: Embracing Life's Possibilities at Every Age

A woman is never too old to chase her dreams, reinvent herself, or start something new. No matter the age, the desire to learn, grow, and explore remains a vital part of who she is. Whether it's pursuing a new career, going back to school, traveling to a place she's always wanted to see, or simply discovering a fresh passion, there's no expiration date on ambition or curiosity. Age does not diminish her ability to create, but instead enriches her with experience, perspective, and resilience. Every year lived adds layers of wisdom and experience that only enhance her ability to contribute in unique and powerful ways.

Emotional growth and self-discovery are lifelong journeys that don't stop with menopause or retirement. A woman can find joy, love, and connection at any stage of life. She can rebuild confidence, nurture new relationships, and redefine what fulfillment means on her own terms. The limitations placed by society's outdated ideas about age have no bearing on the vibrant, purposeful life she can—and deserves to—live every single day.

Conclusion

Age is simply a number, not a limit or a barrier. The truth is, you are never too old to pursue your passions, redefine your purpose, or become the fullest version of yourself. Every year brings new wisdom, new opportunities, and new reasons to keep growing and evolving. The stories society tells about aging are just that — stories. You have the power to rewrite your narrative, to challenge outdated beliefs, and to embrace a life that continues to expand in meaning, joy, and possibility. To stop becoming is simply not an option when you recognize that your journey is far from over.

Choosing to live boldly, curiously, and intentionally at any age is a revolutionary act of self-love and courage. It means stepping beyond fear and cultural expectations to claim the richness that each chapter of life offers. So, no matter where you are in your journey, remember this: your potential doesn't diminish with age — it transforms. Keep dreaming, keep exploring, keep becoming. You are never too old for what matters most — your growth, your happiness, and your light.

Understanding the realities behind aging and menopause empowers us to rewrite the narrative on our own terms. When we separate fact from fiction, we can embrace this phase of life with confidence, curiosity, and even excitement for the growth it offers. This chapter invites you to question the stories you've been told and to recognize the strength, wisdom, and vitality that come with experience. Too old for what? Not for growth, not for purpose, and not for possibility. The becoming never ends—unless we choose to stop. It's about stepping into a mindset that says "no" to limits and "yes" to becoming — because your journey is far from over, and your potential is as boundless as ever.

Affirmation: *"I am not too old; I am just getting started. Every year adds depth, strength, and wisdom to who I am becoming. My journey doesn't expire with age; it expands with purpose."*

Chapter 11

The
Ripple Effect

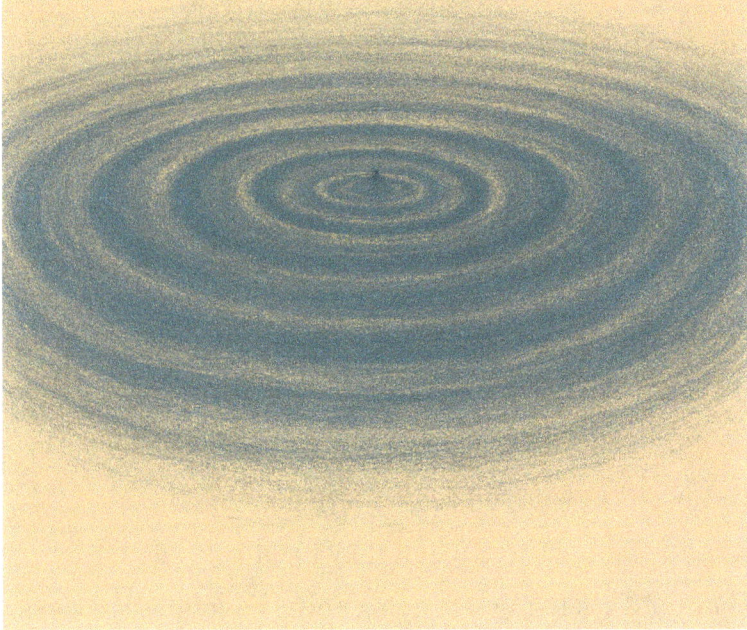

11 The Ripple Effect: When Your Light Touches Others

It is common to feel discouraged and drained during menopause. It can be incredibly difficult to show up for others in a meaningful way. Emotional exhaustion, sadness, or discouragement often leaves you with little energy or capacity to extend support, empathy, or encouragement to those around you. It's not a matter of being selfish or neglectful — it's simply the reality that you can't pour efficiently from an empty cup. When your mind and spirit are weighed down, your instincts to care for others may feel distant or forced, and even small gestures of support can seem overwhelming. A person struggling internally often withdraws — not because they don't care, but because they're trying to survive their own storm.

That's why it's so important to check in with yourself regularly and tend to your own well-being. When you nurture your mental, emotional, and physical health, you position yourself to be more present and supportive to others when they need you. It's not about always being strong or never having tough days — it's about recognizing when you're depleted and giving yourself permission to rest and heal in order to fill your cup. Only then can you return to your relationships and responsibilities with genuine care and renewed strength. Supporting others starts with tending to yourself first, because a healthy, whole heart has so much more to give. When you can thrive through your menopause journey, you will shine, and others will notice as well. When you feel good, you can offer support to someone else — whether it is being active in your community, your church, or whatever it may be. It is always a good feeling when you can give—not for recognition or reward, but simply from the heart.

Pouring Light From an Empty Cup: Two Selves, One Heart

Since I was a little girl, I've always had a heart for helping others. It wasn't something I had to learn or be taught; it felt natural, like it was woven into the very fabric of who I am today. Whether it was comforting a friend, lending a hand to a neighbor, or offering encouragement to someone going through a tough time, I found joy in being a source of support. Looking back, I truly believe this was a gift God intentionally placed within me — a purpose I was meant to carry throughout my life. It's a part of my identity that has shaped my relationships, my work, and the way I move through the world, constantly seeking ways to uplift others, even in seasons when I struggled to uplift myself.

During some of the darkest moments of my menopause journey, I never stopped offering kindness and support to others. But behind the scenes, I was quietly battling my own struggles during my menopause journey. I would show up with a smile, compassion, encouragement, and strength — offering them the support they needed — yet when the doors closed, I faced a very different, private reality, and the emotions I had been suppressing all day started to rise. I wrestled with my insecurities, exhaustion, and unspoken worries — the side of me no one else saw. It's a painful reminder that even the strongest supporters need space to be vulnerable, and that tending to our private struggles is just as important as caring for others. This was exactly what was happening to me. I was giving from a place of emptiness, wearing a smile as a disguise while silently battling my own pain. I thought that if I just kept helping others, it would at least keep anyone from noticing the cracks forming in my spirit. I was offering what little energy I had left because it felt like the only way to keep moving, to feel needed, and to avoid confronting the loneliness of my struggles. But deep down, I knew I was pouring from a nearly dry cup. The more I gave without tending to my pain, the emptier I became.

I was like that split character in the movie Dr. Jekyll and Mr. Hyde. How many of us have been in those shoes? The concept of Dr. Jekyll and Mr. Hyde comes from a classic story about a man who had two very different sides to his personality — one kind, respectable, and well-liked, and the other side was dark, troubled, and hidden from the world. Many of us can relate to this duality, especially when it comes to helping others while silently battling our own struggles. Sometimes, we give our love, kindness, and strength to others while quietly struggling to refill our own reserves. This dual existence—where one of the selves shines brightly for the world, while the other wrestles in silence—is a testament to the resilience and depth of a heart that refuses to give up, even when it feels empty.

The Quiet Power of Giving

There's something extraordinary that happens when you choose to give. Giving is not just about grand gestures or constant sacrifice; it's about allowing your light — however dim it might feel in the moment — to reach someone else's darkness. In those tender, broken places of your journey, your compassion deepens. You begin to see others through a lens of grace because you know what it means to ache in silence. And slowly, as you offer words of encouragement, small acts of kindness, or a simple listening ear, you realize that you're not only lifting others — you're lifting yourself too. Give yourself some credit — even in your brokenness, you're still showing up for others. It's like someone with only a few dollars giving their last to someone in need. You may not have it all together, but you keep giving from the little strength, hope, or light you have. This is the kind of generosity that comes from sacrifice, not surplus, is deeply powerful.

Pouring from a Balanced Cup: Nurturing Yourself While Supporting Others

How do we learn to pour from a balanced cup — neither empty nor overflowing — but just right to sustain us and others? It's about stopping the act behind closed doors and allowing yourself to be both the healer and the one who needs healing. Some may say, how is this even possible without feeling overwhelmed trying to fix me and someone else in the process? It can feel like a tough job, but the key is giving yourself permission to pause. You don't have to hold it all together all the time. Creating space for self-care, asking for support, and practicing compassion for yourself allows you to both give and receive healing without running on empty. It's not about doing it all at once—it's about finding rhythm between pouring out and being refilled. The partner to this is for you to begin to share your story, the cracks in your armor let light flow in and out, sparking connection and courage in others. The more you embrace your truth, the freer you become. When you give with that kind of freedom, it stops being just something you do and becomes part of who you are—a steady light that reaches others not because you have everything figured out, but because you know what it's like to feel lost and still choose to shine for others.

There's a meaningful difference between giving while you're still sitting in darkness and giving after you've started to rise from it. When you give from a place of pain, your kindness often stems from a sense of duty, distraction, or a need for survival. You're pouring from an empty cup, hoping to find a sense of worth or escape in helping others. While it may offer temporary relief or moments of connection, it can also leave you feeling drained and unseen because you're still hiding the parts of yourself that need care and healing. The impact is limited because you're offering what you think others need, not what your whole, honest self has to give.

When you begin to give from a place of healing —
when you've faced your darkness, embraced your
scars, and allowed light back into your life — your
giving changes. It becomes more rooted in wisdom,
empathy, and authenticity. You're no longer seeking
to fill a void within yourself but are now pouring from
a place of overflow. That's when your words carry
weight, your presence calms storms, and your story
inspires others to believe they, too, can rise. The
ripple effect you create when you give from light, not
pain, is deeper, longer-lasting, and transformational
— because it's real, it's whole, and it's fueled by the
strength of someone who's walked through the fire
and still chooses to love.

When I stopped pretending and allowed myself to be
vulnerable and opened up more about my feelings,
everything began to shift. I realized that true giving —
the kind that creates a lasting ripple effect — comes
when you begin to reclaim your light. When I faced my
struggles head-on and found healing in my own
journey, my giving transformed. It became fuller,
richer, and rooted in authenticity. I was no longer

giving to mask my pain but to genuinely lift others—
because I understood their hurt. In that honest space,
I felt peace for the first time in years. I learned that you
can't truly touch the hearts of others if you're afraid to
tend to your own.

The Courage to Take Off the Mask

Coming out of that darkness starts with permission to
admit you're not okay and that you don't have to be
everything for everyone. It begins the moment you stop
hiding behind the mask of "I'm fine" and get honest
with yourself about what you're truly feeling. The first
step isn't some grand, dramatic gesture; it's a quiet
decision to pause, acknowledge your pain, and believe
that you are worthy of peace and healing. This is where
the light starts to break through — in the small, tender
moments when you give yourself grace instead of guilt
and begin to choose yourself in ways you may have
neglected for years.

The Ripple Effect of Sharing Your Story

You create the ripple effect not by waiting until you
have everything figured out, but by choosing to show

up with authenticity and intention in the spaces you occupy right now. It begins with small, genuine acts — a kind word, a heartfelt check-in, a shared story that reminds another woman that they are not alone. When you give from a place of honesty, honoring both your strength and your struggles, it forms a connection that travels further than you'll ever see. Your presence becomes a quiet source of hope, a reminder that even in life's hardest seasons, light can still break through. Every moment you offer encouragement, wisdom, or empathy adds to a wave of healing that reaches far beyond you.

You also create the ripple effect by living in alignment with your truth. When you honor your needs, embrace your growth, and refuse to shrink yourself to meet others' expectations, you quietly permit other women to do the same. Your courage becomes contagious. The way you carry yourself, the choices you make to prioritize your well-being, and the way you uplift others without losing yourself, all send ripples into the lives of those watching — whether they ever say it or not. The ripple effect isn't always about loud, public gestures; it's about the quiet, consistent influence of a woman who chooses to rise — and in doing so, lights the path for others.

This is the ripple effect in motion: when one woman finds the courage to rise, to heal, and to live honestly, it inspires those around her to believe they can too. When you share your journey, you create a ripple effect—your story reaches another woman, offering her hope, courage, and the strength to face her own challenges. One woman's openness can inspire another to speak her truth, creating waves of support that extend far beyond what you can see. Your courage to be vulnerable sends ripples of empowerment that travel from one woman to the next, building a community of strength and understanding. Each story shared is like a pebble dropped in water—its ripples reach far, encouraging women everywhere to rise and thrive together. By embracing and sharing your experience, you become part of a powerful chain reaction that uplifts and transforms the lives of many women beyond your own. Your strength doesn't just stay with you — it touches the people you encounter in ways you may never realize. A simple conversation, a moment of empathy, or your visible resilience becomes a spark for someone else who is quietly struggling. That person, moved by your light, begins to shift their own perspective, making choices that lead to their healing. As they grow stronger, they begin to touch the lives of others in their circle. This is the true ripple effect. One act of light creates waves that move through families, friendships, and communities without end.

What makes this ripple effect so powerful is that it's often unseen but deeply felt. You may never know how many hearts your story, your encouragement, or your presence has reached — but it matters. Every time you show up as your authentic self, you send out waves of strength, hope, and permission for others to do the same. It begins with you, but it never stops with you.

After the ripple effect has taken place, it's important for a woman going through menopause to turn inward and continue tending to her own light. You've poured into others, created connections, and inspired healing;

giving to others is important—but so is keeping your own cup replenished. Remember, life isn't perfect, so your cup may not always be completely full—but it can be balanced. This season of life is still yours to fully embrace. Focus on what brings you joy, rest when your spirit asks for it, and explore new passions or dreams you may have set aside. The ripple you created doesn't mean your work on yourself is finished — it means you've stepped into a new chapter of wisdom and strength, where both giving and receiving are essential.

From there, step into the role of nurturer, mentor, and example for those coming behind you. Use your voice to advocate for conversations around menopause, aging, and emotional wellness. Build communities where women feel seen, valued, and supported. The ripple effect you sparked is not a one-time event; it is an ongoing movement you're now a part of. Keep learning, growing, and sharing your light—not because you have to, but because it feels good to walk fully in your purpose and know your journey is making a lasting difference in the lives of others.

Striving for Balance, Not Perfection

Even after you've created a ripple effect and stepped into your healing, life will still be imperfect. There will be days when old challenges resurface, when exhaustion settles in, or when you find yourself slipping back into old patterns of self-doubt, isolation, or emotional heaviness. That's the reality of this journey—healing isn't a straight line, and menopause, like life, continues to bring seasons of both calm and chaos. It's important to accept that you're human, and moments of struggle don't mean you've failed or lost your light. They simply mean you're alive, navigating a constantly shifting landscape, and learning as you go. When you notice yourself slipping back into those challenges, pause and name what's happening without judgment. Remind yourself of how far you've come and lean back into the practices, people, and truths that pulled you out before. Whether it's journaling, prayer, a walk in nature, a phone call to a trusted friend, or simply sitting with yourself in quiet reflection, return to what grounded you. The key is to respond, not retreat. Life will test you, but your strength is in how quickly you recognize those moments and choose to reach for the light again. That's the real antidote: resilience wrapped in self-compassion.

The Importance of Community

After acknowledging that life is not perfect and setbacks occur, you can emphasize how the community helps sustain the ripple effect. Surrounding yourself with women who uplift, challenge, and hold you accountable is one of the most powerful ways for women to stay grounded when life tries to pull you back into those old patterns. Even one or two authentic connections can help remind you of your light when you forget.

A Reflection Exercise: Trace Your Ripples

Think of one person that you have positively impacted during this season of your life, even if it was a small moment like a kind word or honest conversation. This helps you to see your own significance and reminds you that your light matters. You can frame it as a journal prompt or a quiet moment of reflection to trace the unseen ways you have made a difference.

Remember, the ripple effect is never about perfection or doing everything right — it's about persistence, presence, and the willingness to keep showing up, even when it feels hard. Each time you choose to shine your light, especially through the messiness and uncertainty, you create space for healing, not just for yourself, but for every woman who watches and follows behind. Your journey is a living testament to strength and grace, and with every small act of courage, you weave a tapestry of hope that stretches far beyond what you can see. This is the true power of your light: it doesn't just touch others for a moment; it echoes through generations.

Conclusion

In every season of life, especially through the challenges of menopause, your light holds incredible power — not only to heal yourself but to inspire and uplift those around you. The ripple effect begins when you dare to show up authentically, embracing both your struggles and your strengths. It grows through your willingness to give from a place of truth and self-compassion, knowing that even your smallest acts of kindness can spark hope in someone else's heart. Though life will always bring ups and downs, your choice to keep shining, to keep giving, and to keep healing creates waves that extend far beyond what you can imagine.

As you continue on this journey, remember that your ripple is part of a larger movement — a community of women rising together, lighting the way for each other. There will be moments of setback, and that's okay; it's all part of the imperfect, beautiful process of growth. Keep nurturing your own light, surrounding yourself with support, and celebrating every step forward. Your story, your courage, and your giving will make a lasting difference. The world needs your light — keep letting it shine.

Affirmation: *"As I shine in truth and love, my light creates ripples that reach farther than I can see. I trust that even the smallest act of authenticity can awaken hope, healing, and purpose in someone else's life. Even in my imperfection, my light is worthy, my story matters, and my presence creates ripples of hope and healing in this world."*

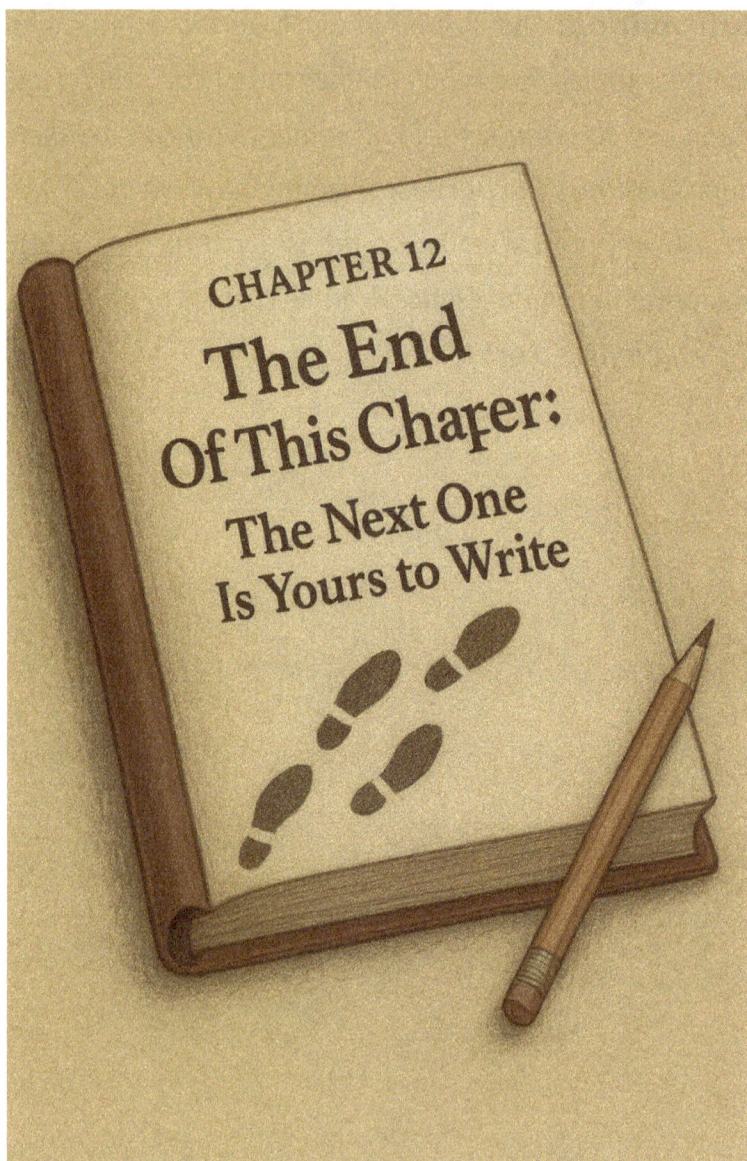

CHAPTER 12

The End
Of This Chapter:
The Next One
Is Yours to Write

12 The End of This Chapter: The Next One is Yours to Write

This is your invitation to walk with intention — to leave behind footprints not just of survival, but of grace, courage, and transformation. Footprints that whisper: I was here. I mattered. I grew. Let this book be a mirror and a map. The mirror that shows you not just who you are, but who you have always been beneath the noise. The map that will guide you through landscapes of doubt and into valleys of rediscovery, where every step reflects your transformation. With every step you take, may you feel more aligned with your truth, more connected to your essence, and more aligned with the life that has been quietly waiting for you to claim it.

The Return to Wholeness

The Return to Wholeness is a profound journey of reclaiming all parts of yourself—mind, body, and soul—after a season of change, challenge, or loss. Especially during menopause, this return invites you to embrace the fullness of who you are, beyond the fluctuations of hormones and the shifting roles life presents. It's about healing old wounds, forgiving yourself for perceived shortcomings, and releasing what no longer serves you. In this sacred process, you move from fragmentation and fatigue toward integration and vitality, rediscovering a deep sense of balance and inner peace that feels both empowering and renewing.

This return is not about perfection or going back to who you once were; it's about stepping into a new, wiser version of yourself with compassion and grace. It calls for patience and gentle self-care, as you rebuild your relationship with your body, nurture your emotional landscape, and reconnect with your spiritual essence. Through this journey, you reclaim your voice, your passions, and your purpose, creating a life that reflects your true, authentic self. The *Return to Wholeness* is a powerful affirmation that no matter the seasons you face, your soul has the strength to heal, grow, and thrive. Keep moving with intention, and trust that nourishing your soul will carry you beyond the footprints of menopause.

Rising Beyond Society's Limits

You are rising. You are stepping into a version of yourself that is wiser, more self-assured, and more unapologetic than ever before. Society feels that your confidence fades, that beauty diminishes, and that self-worth should be questioned, but you have heard and seen the truth: You are stronger now than you have ever been. You carry the wisdom of experience, the freedom of self-acceptance, and the boldness of a woman who refuses to shrink. Menopause may mark the end of one phase of life, but it is not the end of you—it is a new beginning. A moment to step forward with strength, wisdom, and unshakable confidence.

No Longer in the Shadows

You are not the woman you were years ago—you are stronger. You are not meant to stay in the shadows—you are meant to shine. You are not finished—you are just beginning. You have spent years giving, nurturing, and taking care of others, often putting yourself second. But now, it's time to reclaim what has always been yours: your confidence, self-worth, and undeniable strength. The doubts you once had no longer hold power over you. They don't define you. The changes? They don't diminish you. The world may tell you to shrink, to quiet down, to fade into the background, but you know better. You have proven, time and time again, that resilience lives within you. You have embraced change, honored your journey, and refused to settle for anything less than the bold, empowered woman you were meant to be.

The Strength in Seeking Support

Never be afraid to seek support. There is profound strength in reaching out, in allowing yourself to be held, heard, and supported. Too often, we're taught to wear resilience like armor — to push through silently, to carry the weight alone. But true empowerment comes not from isolation, but from connection. Seeking support is not stepping back — it's stepping forward with wisdom, grace, and the courage to say, I matter enough to be cared for. Let that be your reminder: you are worthy of support, and it's always okay to ask for it.

Walking This Journey Together

Though this is the final chapter of the book, as you step into your next chapter beyond these pages, know that I am stepping into mine as well. I remain committed to walking this path — not just beside you, but with you, because transformation is not a solo act. It's a shared rhythm and a rising together. This book is not just a reflection of your journey — it is a reflection of mine as well. It carries my footprints and my stories. My soul has traveled this journey with you, not as a distant voice, but as a companion, a witness, and a fellow traveler. Every word in these pages has been written from a place of deep empathy, lived experience, and unwavering belief in my power to reclaim and reshape my own destiny.

This chapter may be coming to a close, but my journey and hopefully yours don't end here either. I, too, will continue forward with renewed strength, deeper resilience, and a heart that has been shaped by the same winds of change. I, too, have faced the questions, the quiet reckonings, and the moments of doubt and discovery—and I walk this journey alongside you, step by step toward rising. I will continue to show up — in words, in rituals, in reflections — offering my guidance to light the way. My purpose is rooted in helping women like you rediscover your brilliance, reclaim your voice, and reimagine what's possible beyond the confines of society's expectations.

No Looking Back—Only Forward

Walking forward means embracing this truth, shedding limitations, and finally allowing yourself to take up space unapologetically. It means standing tall, speaking your truth, and knowing—deep in your soul—that you are enough, exactly as you are. There comes a moment when looking back no longer serves the soul—when nostalgia becomes noise and regret no longer holds you down. You were never meant to live in reverse. The call now is forward — into the parts of you not yet explored, but well within your power to navigate. Let what's behind you be the soil that grew your strength, not the anchor that holds you. With every challenge, you are being shaped into someone stronger, wiser, and more radiant. So, when the skies darken and the winds howl, lift your eyes and see the possibilities ahead. Trust that God is carrying you even when you can't see the path. The storms will pass — and when it does, you'll find yourself standing in a new light, with testimony etched into your soul and a deeper knowing of just how far you've come.

Taking Action: From Inspiration to Real Results.

While this book was meant to inspire and uplift women through the menopause journey, it is more than just a source of encouragement. True transformation happens when knowledge meets action. Don't let this book sit unread on your shelf or remain only an idea in your mind. The insights shared here are tools — designed to educate, guide, and empower you to make real changes in your life. This is where the true healing begins: when you take what you've learned and apply it, step by step, to reclaim your energy, balance, and confidence. Inspiration lights the path, but action is what carries you forward.

Walking with Purpose: Writing the Next Chapter of Your Life

Now, the real question is: How will you write the next chapter of your story? Will you step forward boldly, embracing life with joy and confidence? Will you own your power, knowing that you are enough, just as you are? This next chapter begins not with certainty, but with courage—and you are choosing to rise.

You have spent years growing, evolving, and adapting—and this journey is proof that you are capable of more than you ever imagined. The challenges you've faced, the doubts you've overcome, and the resilience you've built have led you to this very moment. And now, you get to decide how the next chapter unfolds.

As you continue your journey beyond the footprints of menopause, know that challenges may still arise — but they no longer define you. You've already walked through fire and emerged with wisdom etched into your soul. The road ahead may bring new questions, unexpected turns, or moments that test your patience, but now, you carry tools forged in transformation: self-compassion, clarity, and the quiet knowing that you have faced hard things before — and you have risen. You are no longer walking blindly; you are walking with intention, with a deeper understanding of your worth, and with the courage to meet each challenge as an opportunity for growth.

You will move forward not because life is easy, but because you are ready. Ready to honor your truth. Ready to choose yourself. Ready to rewrite the story when old narratives try to return. Each step you take is a declaration: I am here. I am evolving. I am enough. When the winds shift or the path grows steep, you will pause, breathe, and remember that you are not alone. You are part of a collective of women rising — each one leaving behind footprints of resilience, grace, and transformation. So, keep walking, keep trusting, and allow yourself to grow with each step. The journey is yours, and you are more than equipped to meet it.

This chapter may end here, but your story does not. The future is not written for you. You are the author. You hold the pen. What do you want to say? So go forth boldly, brilliantly, unapologetically YOU. You've earned this moment — not just through the challenges you've faced, but through the grace with which you've risen. You are no longer defined by what others expect or what the world once told you to be. You are defined by your truth, your light, and your unwavering commitment to becoming the fullest version of yourself. Boldness doesn't mean being loud; it means being clear. Brilliance doesn't mean perfection; it means shining from within. Being unapologetically you means standing in your story without shrinking, without editing, without asking for permission.

This is your time to take up space, to speak with power, and to live with intention. Let your presence be a declaration of everything you've survived and everything you're stepping into. Let your choices reflect your values, your joy, and your sacred knowing. You don't need to explain your glow or justify your journey. You are here to embody it — fully, fiercely, and freely. So go forth with your head high and your heart open. The world needs your voice, your vision, and your vibrance. And most of all, you need you — whole, radiant, and walking forward without apology. The future is not handed to you; it's written by you, one brave word at a time. Pen in hand, truth in heart, and fire in soul—this is what a true author looks like.

Through this journey, you have rediscovered your voice, reclaimed your self-worth, and stood firm in your power. You have walked through uncertainty, only to find that your strength has always been within you—waiting for you to fully embrace it. So, as you move forward, know this: You are not alone. I am still here. Still walking. Still growing. Still believing. Together, we will leave footprints that speak of courage, compassion, and rebirth. Together, we shape a future that honors every version of who we've been — and celebrates every possibility of who we're becoming.

Now step forward unapologetically—no longer bound by fear, no longer questioning your value. You own your beauty, your wisdom, and your resilience.

As we reach the final page of this book, we arrive at a pause, not an ending, but a gentle breath before the next step. The road doesn't end here. It simply curves out of sight, waiting for you to continue walking it with renewed strength, deeper wisdom, a straighter path, and a heart wide open to possibilities.

I hoped these chapters offered more than surface-level reading but invited deeper reflection, emotional resonance, and a stirring call to rise. I hope they have stirred something sacred within you — something motivational, spiritual, and profoundly uplifting. To me, *Beyond the Footprints of Menopause* means that every past footprint matters—both the struggles and the victories—but the true beauty lies in choosing to leave new ones that reflect growth, strength, and possibility. May the stories, reflections, and rituals within the pages of this book, *Beyond the Footprints of Menopause,* leave you feeling truly seen, deeply heard, and lovingly held.

Close this chapter with grace, but don't close the door to what's ahead. Step beyond the footprints of menopause, carrying your wisdom and strength, and embrace the limitless possibilities that await you. You are already on your way. Remember to be a source of encouragement to others—God bless!

Lifetime Affirmation: *"Though this chapter closes, my story rises—I walk forward not with uncertainty, but with courage. I am not defined by endings but empowered by beginnings. "The road ahead bows to* *my boldness. I trust my steps, even when I can't yet see the path."*

From My Heart to Yours

This menopause journey has
shaped the woman I have become,
With strength and grace, I'm never done.

Each step I take, I make my mark,
A light that glows beyond the dark.
Each step I take, I find my way,
A brighter path, a clearer day.

No longer bound by fear or flaws,
I move ahead and embrace my own
cause.

Now step into your power, embrace
what's true,
This journey shines, and so can you.

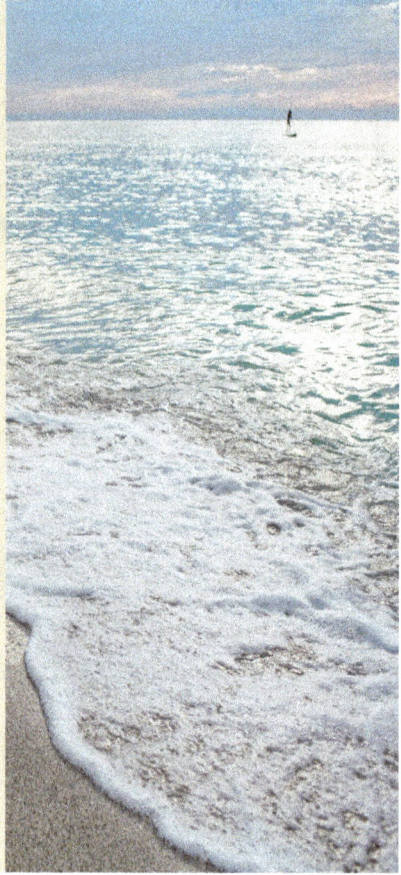